# THE GOOD-TIME FITNESS BOOK

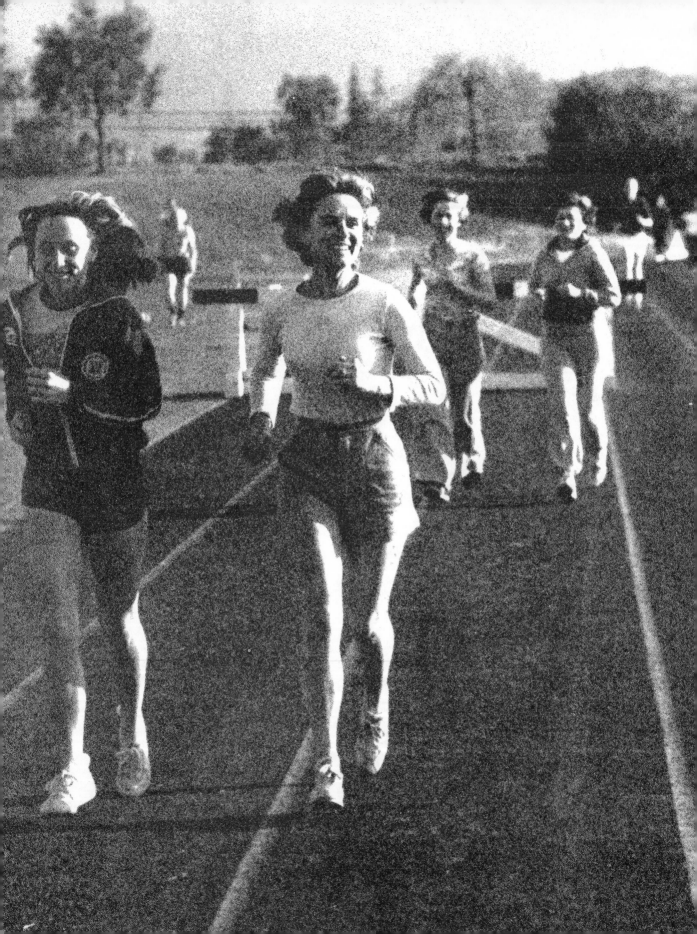

# THE GOOD-TIME FITNESS BOOK

## THOMAS FAHEY

### PHOTOGRAPHS BY
### WAYNE GLUSKER

Butterick Publishing

To Kilty, my wife and training partner;
my mother, the ageless jock; and my father,
the exception.

**Library of Congress Cataloging in Publication Data**
Fahey, Thomas D.
   The good-time fitness book.

   1.   Physical fitness.   I.   Title.
GV481.F27      613.7'1      78-55745
ISBN 0-88421-059-6

Printed in United States of America

Book Design: Ron Shey

Although sports and physical activity generally have a positive effect on your health, they are not without risk and it is, therefore, suggested that you consult with your doctor prior to the commencement of any exercise program. The author and publisher of this book assume no responsibility or liability for injury resulting from your exercise program or any activities suggested in this book.

# FOREWORD

In my profession I am occasionally called upon to lecture to groups of the general public on physical fitness. Fitness, what is it, how to achieve it and maintain it are questions of ever increasing interest. My experience with giving lectures is to leave plenty of time for questions and answers. It is unfortunate that while physical fitness is a quality almost universally admired, it is also a state of human experience which is also frequently misunderstood. In discussing fitness I find myself having to correct generally held, but false impressions. Often, I have been asked to recommend an understandable book which the average person could consult on the whys and hows of fitness. Since the first time I was unable to answer that question, I have felt the need for a guide to fitness such as THE GOOD-TIME FITNESS BOOK. In his book Dr. Fahey has provided us with an interestingly written, simple to follow, and scientifically based program of fitness. Written in the contemporary idiom, and presented in a format people will enjoy reading and be able to relate to, Dr. Fahey describes why and how to exercise, how to begin exercising, where to find help and meet people, and common pitfalls and misconceptions of exercise. In many ways exercise programs are like diets; the programs are usually successful so long as they are adhered to. Unfortunately the diets and exercise programs frequently fail as they are not followed. In making the active lifestyle the basis of his exercise program, Dr. Fahey describes how purpose and enjoyment become the means as well as the ends of the program. It is my belief that this total exercise program can contribute to making you a more attractive, effective, happy, and vigorous person.

George A. Brooks, Ph.D.

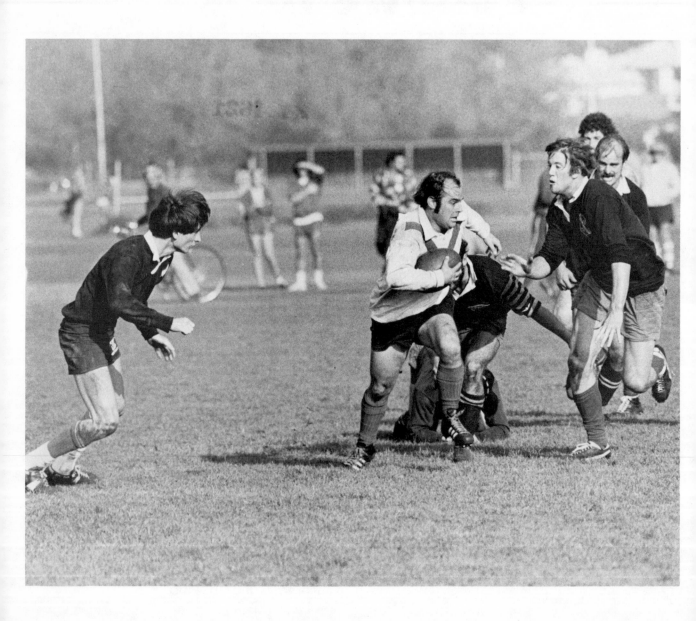

# PREFACE

**W**e all secretly admire the person who has a well-tanned, lean, and graceful body and seems to be equally at home on the tennis court, track, ski slope, or dance floor. This individual seems tireless and able to attack every activity with vitality and enthusiasm. I have chosen to call this man or woman the "Total Jock." The "Total Jock" is in harmony with his body and has learned to skillfully utilize his full potential by involvement in a variety of sports and exercises that are done for their own sake.

The aim of the "Total Jock" program is to make exercise fun by making sports and physical activity an important part of your life rather than a drudgery used to prevent a heart attack ten or 15 years from now. Only by involving yourself in a variety of physical experiences that you enjoy can you ever expect to stay on a lifetime exercise program. You will learn how to use your body in more ways than running in a straight line for 20 minutes or lifting a weight off your chest. The "Total Jock" will systematically develop total fitness with strength, endurance, and flexibility exercises, and involvement in a variety of sports that teach you to use your whole body.

The "Total Jock" takes a little more time than most popular exercise programs, but the results are much greater. By becoming a jock you will begin to lead the active life and experience its benefits: a more attractive body, better control over your own movement, success in sports such as skiing, and a faster, more exciting lifestyle.

I have designed this program in response to the needs of people I have counseled in my exercise physiology laboratory. These people expressed the desire for a complete fitness program that would develop

7

strength as well as endurance and allow them to win at sports or at least enjoy sports. We have adapted the physical and psychological techniques of professional and world-class athletes in designing the "Total Jock" program. I am convinced that if you are willing to put in the time, you can become the "Total Jock." It is within your reach!

Photo courtesy of Coast Catamaran, Irvine, California.

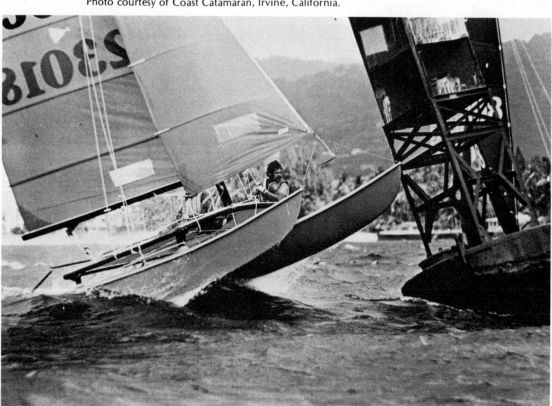

# CONTENTS

# INTRODUCTION

**I** am the director of the De Anza Human Physiology Laboratory, an ultrasophisticated fitness diagnostic center in California. We study and design exercise programs for people ranging from world-class and professional athletes to the physically disabled. Our services include evaluation of body fat and muscle mass, muscle strength assessment, measurement of blood fats, and computerized analysis of the heart, lungs, and muscular systems during exercise on a treadmill. Detailed physical fitness profiles are prepared and exercise programs designed that help people achieve the maximum improvement with the least amount of risk and discomfort. In addition, the laboratory has become a community resource center where questions of all kinds can be answered about exercise and sports.

Unfortunately, most people don't have access to a modern sports medicine laboratory to help them with their exercise training or to answer questions about exercise physiology. I wrote this book to fill the gap between a modern fitness diagnostic center and the numerous self-help exercise books presently flooding the market. Many books on the subject are inadequate because

1. They are often written by people with little knowledge of exercise physiology. The information imparted is often inaccurate.
2. They attempt to capitalize on the "get something for nothing attitude" by recommending inadequate exercise programs that require a minimum time commitment.
3. They stress only one component of fitness, such as strength or

endurance, instead of the development of a body fit for a variety of movement experiences.

4. They take the fun out of training, presenting a "fire and brimstone" scenario of imminent death by heart attack if you don't jog.

I am advocating a sports-oriented lifestyle in this book. Sports and fitness become a part of your life because you love them. Possible protection from heart disease is an added benefit; it comes with the territory. I have presented guidelines for getting started and improving once you get into the fitness process. I stress well-rounded physical fitness. Endurance, strength, flexibility, speed, and sports skills are required for the active life.

I have tried to answer many of the common questions about exercise physiology and training. I have provided you with the basics of how the body responds to exercise and how to develop fitness that will make you capable of reacting to a variety of situations.

There are many levels of sport. You can get the same enjoyment from exercise that the pros do. You may not be able to hit a tennis ball as hard as they do at Wimbledon or shoot baskets like the New York Knicks, but you can be just as serious and dedicated. All levels of sport are similar—people competing against themselves to get better. "Winning" in sports means performing up to your expectations.

# CHAP1TER

# YOU CAN BE A JOCK

**66T**oday I ran two miles in 16 minutes; that's 15 miles this week," panted a sweaty, tired looking woman running in San Francisco's Golden Gate Park. "At this rate, I should live to be a hundred." The woman ran off, deciding to plod along for another mile or so. Across town at a health spa with the latest rage in weight lifting machines, a man was also working on physical fitness. "Fifteen, 16, 17 . . . that's it," grimaced a heavyset man as he strained to squeeze out the last few reps on a leg press machine. "This stuff is miserable, but I get one hell of a workout in only 30 minutes."

Each of these people is typical of men and women throughout the country. They are involved in boring exercise routines. Why? Because they desperately want physical fitness and all of its benefits: an attractive body, better health, and an active lifestyle. These people have different methods, but very similar goals. Each method appeals to an individual temperament and body type.

The jogger was lean in stature and very methodical about her program. She expected a regular decrease in her running times and at least ten years added to her life span because of all the work she did. The weight lifter was different. He had big muscles, but also a protruding beer belly. The jogger was trying to keep from having a heart attack, while the weight lifter was trying to develop big muscles so he would look physically fit. Neither person had developed well-rounded physical fitness. Their programs were narrow, concentrating on only certain parts of their bodies. Although strength training and running are important components of physical fitness, they were both chasing an illusion that really was not that important to either of them. Both people had one thing in common: They were not enjoying what they were doing.

From my experience as an exercise consultant, I would say that both of these people are likely to quit their training programs within a couple of months. Why? Because neither one really had a good reason to continue exercising. The heart attack the runner is trying to prevent doesn't seem real. A seemingly distant event such as a possible heart attack usually can't hold a person to a training program that is exhausting and not enjoyable. The weight lifter will find that he will have to work pretty hard to get those big muscles. He'll ask himself, "Is a little muscle worth all this boring work I have to do in this sweaty gym?" These people will probably fail because they are not having fun, and the results do not appear to be worth the effort.

Many people seem to thrive on exercise. They look good in bathing suits, and they always seem to be enjoying themselves. They are constantly off skiing, playing tennis, climbing mountains, or hitting a softball. They always seem to be involved in sports or some form of exercise. These people are the jocks. Exercise and sports are an important part of their life.

Why is it that the jocks don't seem to have the same problem staying on an exercise program and staying in shape that the rest of us do?

1. Jocks exercise because they like to.
2. Jocks do endurance and strength exercises to help them in their other sports.
3. Distant goals, such as protection against heart disease, are secondary to more immediate goals, such as having a good time.

The "Total Jock" has an adventurous, young approach to life. The "Total Jock" program seeks to develop total physical fitness by making sports participation an important part of your life. Little by little you will be introduced to new activities. You will become proficient in several sports and develop an exercise program that is centered around these new pursuits. Fitness will be easy because you will be doing what you like and having fun.

Jocks are more successful with their fitness programs than most of us because they do it for fun. They do many of the more tedious types of training, such as running and strength training, for a purpose: exercises help them play. Sports and games are played for their own sake. They experience playing tennis, skiing powder, and playing racquetball as part of life's great pleasures, not as medicine to prevent heart attacks. They look good on the beach because their active lives keep them fit and attractive. Jocks lead a fast, active life that gives them nice bodies and an active outlook on life. For them physical fitness is not something grudgingly worked on but the natural result of a vigorous and enjoyable way of living.

I think you can become a jock. You can become exceedingly fit by getting hooked on a more active lifestyle. The "Total Jock" program

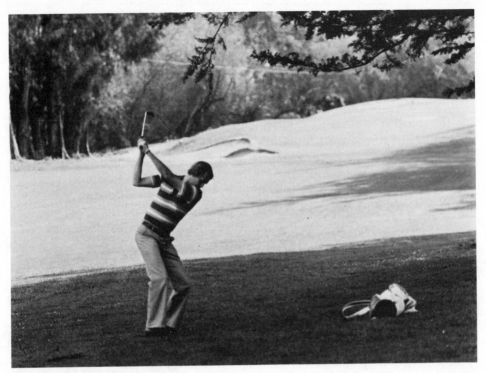
Improved fitness may help your golf game.

will help you develop a whole new repertoire of fun things to do. You have the time, and if you don't, you can make time. With a little effort you can improve, and with a little more effort you can be good! Involvement in sports will help make you totally fit for two reasons: (1) You will enjoy what you are doing. (2) You will have a purpose for running and strength training—to help you improve in the sports you have come to love.

Enjoyment and purpose are the keys to this approach. Recently, a man came into my laboratory to check on his fitness level. In one year he had lost 30 pounds of fat, increased his strength considerably, and greatly improved his treadmill performance. I asked him, "What did you do, buy a house in the middle of the running track?"

"No," he said, "I got a divorce. Now that I'm single again, I have to be ready for the chase."

This man had a purpose: to renew the old sex appeal or suffer possible rejection. Physicians in family practice will tell you that patients who suddenly lose a great deal of weight after years of unsuccessful diets are often contemplating a change in—or are in the process of changing—their personal relationships. If you can develop a purpose, you can do wonders with your fitness program. I think developing skills in a number of sports is probably more satisfactory than divorce, but I'll let you be the judge of that.

Let's put fun and excitement into your program. Look at sports and games the way you look at food. Have you ever wondered why so many people are overweight? Everyone knows that being fat is not healthy, but the fear of fat is not as great as the pleasure of eating a big piece of chocolate cake. Pleasure and immediate gratification will win out every time over more noble motives. Similarly, you are fighting a losing battle if you exercise only because it's good for you. When you train for fun, and exercise is part of your life, your program will be easy to stay on. When exercise is a pleasure, it's a piece of cake.

Make a game of it. Have you ever watched a bunch of kids at a swimming pool? They are usually involved in some kind of game that they've made up. Kids seem to be always moving and active. When you get a little older, you seem to spend a lot more time lying around the pool deck.

You've got to get psyched! Play water volleyball, underwater relays, 42-man squamish, or any other game you can make up. Play, and you'll be developing your fitness without even thinking about it.

## THE TOTAL JOCK: FIVE HOURS A WEEK IN THE FAST LANE

When I was a kid, I used to read *Superman Magazine*, the 1950's version of the bionic man and woman. Inside the comic book, Charles Atlas, the granddaddy of strong men, always had a full-page advertisement. He was dressed in a hokey-looking leopard skinned suit and had huge ripply muscles and a beautiful girl sitting on each shoulder. The ad also showed a cartoon of a 98-pound wimp who got sand kicked in his face. After he completed the Charles Atlas course, he came back to the beach and wasted the bully who had previously abused and embarrassed him. Already very interested, I read on: "Check the kind of body you want"

☐ A Massive Chest      ☐ A More Exciting Life
☐ Bull Neck      ☐ Win at Sports
☐ Dynamic Personality      ☐ Endless Endurance
☐ Washboard Stomach

All the kids I knew checked every one of the boxes. We understood intuitively that there was more to fitness than any one of these factors. We knew that endurance, strength, flexibility, and speed were all desirable. Why is it then that so many people have a one-box physical fitness program? Unless you can use your body, you are not physically fit. Limited exercise programs solely involving running or strength training only promote the illusion of fitness. But like the automobile manufacturers who produce imitations of the Cadillac, they fool no one. There are so many fun sports to do. All you have to do is get hooked.

Practical-minded people often can't relate to a sports-centered lifestyle. How do you describe searching the ocean depths with a scuba tank, skiing in waist-deep powder, or slamming a devastating cross-court backhand. Not only do you develop physical fitness doing these things, but you get a tremendous rush. My wife and I recently vacationed with another couple in Hawaii, where we experienced a sort of tropical decathlon. Every day we surfed, ran, played tennis, or went scuba diving—great contrasts to the night life made both more enjoyable. The highlight of the vacation was a big-game fishing trip. My friend hooked a 50-pound Mahi Mahi. He struggled for over 45 minutes to land that fish. Catching it took every ounce of strength in his body. He would gain several feet of line only to lose it in an instant. Finally the fish jumped into the air in a brilliant display of color and raw power. My friend had always thought that I was crazy for spending every last nickel I made skiing. I think after catching that fish, he realized that no price could be put on physical experience involving the total being. Jocks stay fit so sports experiences can be enjoyed. If you are not fit, you will be panting for air on the tennis court and lose. You won't enjoy the sports that are important to you. Running and strength exercises are a lot easier when you know they are necessary for success in the activities that you love.

I have observed that the best athletes naturally follow the "Total Jock" program. Why is it that they can train long hours for so long and never seem to get tired of it? Bruce Jenner trained for more than 12 years, enduring personal and financial hardship, to win the gold medal in the decathlon, and yet his goal kept him going. Yes, the Olympic championship and its rewards were obviously valuable to him. But the process of achieving the goal was just as enjoyable. To the jock, involvement in sport is a pleasure. John Powell, discus medalist and former world record holder, said to me, "I see my sport as an art form. It's something I have become totally engrossed in." Powell's love of discus throwing, an event that takes only one second to perform, has turned him into a totally fit man. Not only does he have great strength and endurance, but he has tremendous control over his body. Watching a skier like Suzy Chaffee, you see a combination of beauty, endurance, strength, agility, and grace. These athletes don't mind endurance and strength exercises because they lead to better performance.

You are really no different from the champion athlete. You, too, can develop a high degree of fitness by involvement in many sports. The essence of competition is to improve yourself. This is true at both the highest and lowest levels of competition. Remember, the jogger of today can surpass the performances of many champions of a century ago. It's all relative. You are on a continuum with the athlete.

The top athletes I know of use other activities to help them in their specialties. Arnold Schwarzenegger, the great body builder, practices ballet to help him to move gracefully. Most professional football players use games like handball and basketball to develop quick feet. Because the strength and endurance exercises are part of their overall lifestyle, they become fun. They now have an immediate purpose. To a jock, taking six months off from a training program has a much more immediate effect than the vague possibility of a heart attack 15 years from now. The deconditioned jock can't get the job done. Your lungs burn when you try to ski down the hill, thus forcing you into the bar several hours early. Your lack of condition puts you one step away from getting the shot that separates the winners and losers. You get that old feeling in your bones. Now that's incentive for staying on your program.

During a lecture I gave to one of my fitness groups, a lady in her early 60's said to me, "I haven't got the energy to play golf any more, and I love that game. I just can't seem to make it around the course without feeling dead." Although golf doesn't require extreme stamina, poorly conditioned people will get sore feet after 18 holes. A tired player can't perform consistently; a well-rounded fitness program is necessary for success. I convinced the woman that a regular schedule of walking, jogging, and strength exercises would help her golf game. She started a regular routine and has remained on it ever since, over a year and a half. She told me that not only has her golf game improved, but she feels better and has more pep.

A 35-year-old woman came into my laboratory recently for advice about an exercise program that was appropriate for her age. "My doctor told me now that I'm getting older, I should start doing things suited to my age." She wanted to be old. She rejected any program that involved sports, jogging, or anything else vigorous. She was young and healthy, yet she was ready for the rocking chair. Franklyn Pennock is the world record holder in the high jump for men over 70 years old and a total jock. He said, "I would rather be dead than not be able to be in sports."

He was on his way to practice throwing the discus and javelin in preparation for the world seniors track and field championship in Europe. That 35-year-old woman was older than Franklyn Pennock in a lot of ways. All you're going to get from a rocking chair is splinters.

## GO FOR IT!

My friend and I stood on the edge of a cornice overlooking the west face of KT-22 in Squaw Valley, one of the steepest ski runs in North America. He stood there for about five minutes, petrified. I called out, "Let's go; rest on the chair!"

Finally, I skied over to him to find out what the trouble was. "Damn, this thing is steep," he gasped.

"Look, you're going to have to get down somehow. You have the ability. That mountain isn't going anywhere no matter how long you look at it. Go for it! Point your skis down the hill and keep turning."

He timidly stemmed his ski down the fall line and made a turn. He then slid around a giant mogul for a perfectly executed move. Down the hill he went, until finally he was at the bottom. He didn't have to hesitate; he could have done it right away.

You don't have to hesitate either. All those fun sports that other people do are there for your enjoyment. All you have to do is follow a few simple suggestions. Learn to dream a little. Dreaming is part of your fitness program. Dreaming about skiing, surfing, backpacking, and tennis will help you do your endurance and strength exercises. As Thoreau said, "When I see a person young or old, rich or poor, who has a realizable dream for which he is willing to exchange a piece of his life, I know that person is building toward the highest goal. He is rising to a new level of being, raising his precious will to become stronger, braver, maybe even kinder and wiser."

## THE "TOTAL JOCK" PROGRAM

The "Total Jock" process is simple. You develop skills in a variety of sports that you enjoy. Endurance, strength, and flexibility exercises are practiced in support of your sports. Although each person's program will be slightly different, the results will be the same—an active lifestyle, well-rounded physical fitness, an attractive body, an improved self-image, and greater self-confidence. You won't have to develop physical fitness grudgingly any longer because exercise will be fun. This program will show you how to get started and how to progress. Anyone can do it!

These are some guidelines for beginning this program:

1. Don't be afraid to try something new.
2. Don't be self-conscious. Learn to compete against yourself. Success in competitive games will come with your developing competence.
3. Be patient. We all progress at different rates. Don't worry about results that seem to be too slow. Enjoy the process of being a "Total Jock." The process is what separates this exercise program from the others.
4. Be realistic. The best the "Total Jock" can promise is a fit body, not a part in a movie.

## PART OF YOUR LIFESTYLE

Every day people tell me why they want to exercise. Sometimes I have to read between the lines, but several reasons are expressed by most people:

1. They want to feel better and be healthier.
2. Exercise is fun.
3. Exercise helps to improve sports performance.
4. They want to look better and have more sex appeal.
5. Exercise helps them to socialize.

All these reasons are certainly valid, but how many people have exercise programs that do any of these things? Many types of programs are popular today. Some people practice ineffective 30-minutes-per-week, low-intensity exercise programs. Others prefer health spa weight lifting programs. Some are into marathon training. Most of these programs are inadequate because they aren't strenuous enough, or emphasize only one system of the body.

Several exercise programs have been popularized recently because they require very little time. They claim to produce physically fit people in as little as 12 hours of training. These programs may produce fitness by nursing home standards, but not by the standards of the vast majority of exercise scientists and physicians. Fitness means a lot more effort than picking turnips in the garden more vigorously or pushing the vacuum cleaner harder.

It surprises me how many people equate a good figure or big muscles with physical fitness. I agree with Dr. Ken Cooper, author of the best-seller *Aerobics,* that "You can live without an attractive body, but you can't live without a healthy cardiovascular system." Strength exercises do very little to develop your heart, lungs, and metabolism. If you have to choose between types of exercises, then pick endurance. But why choose? A nice body is important, too. By combining strength exercises with endurance activities, you can be healthy and look healthier. Combine firm and well-toned muscles with the ability to keep on going. You'll have more fun that way.

I don't think that there are many shortcuts. Your fitness program will succeed only if it is interwoven in your life fabric. The "Total Jock" doesn't take that much time. Roger Bannister broke the four-minute mile with 45 minutes of training per day, but they were quality minutes. If you have an organized training routine, you can finish the endurance and strength efforts and have more time available for the fun part of the program—sports and games.

Find other people to play with. Your program is a lot easier if you do it with other people. You don't need to own a cabin to go skiing. Go in with 15 people, and the price comes down. Go down and hit a tennis ball against a wall, and pretty soon you'll have a game. Borrow a friend's camping gear, and take off for a weekend. Jog with a friend. One of the best ways to get involved in a new activity is by taking a class. You will mingle with people who are also starting out. Classes will give you a chance to sample a lot of sports and learn the fundamentals. There are thousands of people out there who would love to do some of these sports with you. Go out and meet them.

## THE FEMALE JOCK

During the past several Olympics, the world has been enchanted by the women's gymnastics competitions. The athletes have exhibited strength, flexibility, and incredible athletic ability and at the same time have presented themselves with beauty and grace. This positive image of physically fit women has done much to increase the participation of the average American woman in sports and exercise. Recent legislation has made it possible for women to gain equal access to athletic fields and to

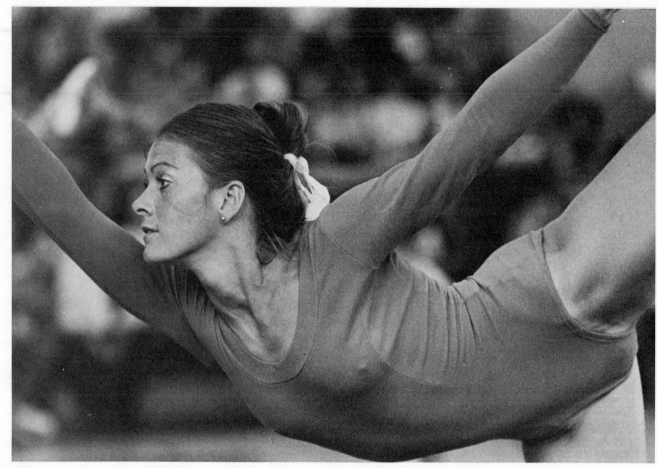

In the past several Olympics, the world has been enchanted by women's gymnastics competition.

receive an important part of their education—the opportunity to participate in sports and physical activity.

I think we are beginning to move past the time when a physically
fit woman is not considered feminine. Women don't have to be closet
exercisers anymore. Now there are almost as many female jocks as male
jocks. (You don't have to wear one to be one.) A woman who can ski,
play tennis, and join in a volleyball game is much more appealing than
one who is afraid to mess up her hair by going swimming.

Physiologists are finding that the gap in performance levels
between the sexes is not as great as was once thought. Women can do
any sport they want. Our school systems have in the past denied

adequate exposure to jock sports to most women. I think that for this reason women are more timid about trying new sports and activities. This program is a natural for women. Once you try some of these new fun things to do, you will become hooked. Your total fitness program will be easy. Many women jog. How about adding a sport? You will be amazed at the effect of adding a weekly racquetball game to your fitness and weight control program. And if you're worried about getting large, bulky muscles, forget it. Unless you are taking shots of male hormones, exercise will only firm up your muscles, not build them up.

## THE YOUNG JOCK

A 15-year-old boy recently came to see me for exercise counseling. "I'll do anything to get into shape. I don't want to be dog meat this season." *Dog meat* is an expression used by some football coaches to describe third-string players. The dog meat do little playing and act as tackling dummies for the first string. We are taught very early that if you are not a winner, you should retire. I spend a lot of time convincing parents that it doesn't matter if their child can't make the Olympic team, but it does matter if the child doesn't develop love of sport and exercise. I hate to see a child burned out about sports at 14. Too many parents and coaches try to live through young people. Sports should be a positive experience. Too often, organized sports destroy any physiological benefits by causing psychological trauma.

The "Total Jock" should be a family affair. Children should be encouraged to jog along with the rest of the family. Sports skills should be taught at a young age. Early development of sports skills will make lifetime fitness a snap. Concentrate on developing your children's positive attitudes about sports and fitness rather than on developing unhappy little athletic robots.

Play is a spontaneous activity in children. Unfortunately, it is often suppressed by the dictates of adults. Judy Reeder Calpin, a 1964 Olympian and presently a swim coach, said, "You wouldn't believe the pressure that some parents put on their children to succeed. At the Santa Clara Swim Club, one day of practice a week was set aside for parents' observation. Swimmers who just the day before were having a great time appeared to be on the verge of nervous breakdown when the parents were watching." If your children are in athletics, make sure that sports are for them and not for you.

In the United States, not enough emphasis is placed on mass participation. Several countries in Europe have been extremely successful in international athletics in recent years because they involve a majority of the population in sports. In America we have an even greater opportunity because of our affluence and mobility. Make the effort. You and your family can improve your fitness by greater involvement in sports together.

## GET PSYCHED!

There is no such thing as an instant athlete. Success in sports is built upon small steps. Say to yourself, "I can be better." Constantly think of ways to improve your fitness and sports skills. The secret of sports success is self-image and good fundamentals. When you have these, you will improve in leaps and bounds. I have seen amazing changes in the most unlikely people. Karen looked like a human Mack truck when she came to me for exercise counseling. Although she was only 34 years old, almost 40 percent of her body weight was fat. Her metabolism resembled that of someone 30 years older. In short, she was a physical wreck. She made up her mind that she was going to fit into the dress she wore in college, a size ten. At first she struggled; exercise was difficult and painful, but she made progress. I asked her to keep a log so she could follow her improvement. The pounds melted away. A funny thing happened to her—she got hooked on a sport: aerobic dance. She didn't mind dancing; in fact, she didn't even consider it exercise. Within eight months after joining the dance group, she could fit into her college dress. She looked like a different person: slim, energetic, and graceful. Karen had a goal that was important to her. She believed in herself. When she got hooked on a pleasurable activity, she made the greatest progress. Her self-confidence improved almost immediately. Karen now believes anything is possible. Her life had expanded at the same time her fat was disappearing.

You can have sports success, too, if you establish reasonable short term goals. As soon as you achieve one goal, establish another. Let's say that you can't make it around the track once. Your goal will be to jog one of the straightaways. After you do this, tell yourself that you can jog 50 yards further. Before you know it, you will make it around the whole track. Don't think so much about what you can or can't do now. Think about what you are going to do.

You say that you've never climbed a mountain? Start by hiking up

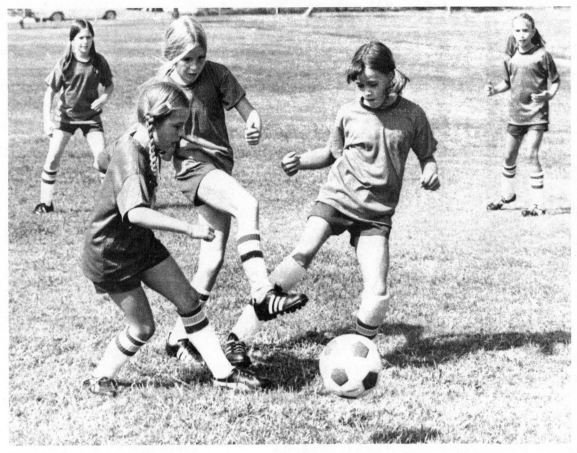
Encourage children to enjoy sports.

a hill; then climb something a little more difficult. Pretty soon you will climb a mountain. Above all, enjoy the process. What's the use of having a long life if your life is dull? The "Total Jock" is exciting. Get psyched and become optimistic.

All those people who look so good skiing down the hill or defeating everyone on the tennis court are no different from you. They made a commitment to success in something that they learned to love. Maybe you'll never jump off of a cornice at Squaw Valley, but you can lead a more expanded lifestyle. Don't let life pass you by. Experience the satisfaction of physical participation. Start to see yourself as an active, dynamic person who experiences things. Don't be a spectator. An exercise program that is part of your life is easy to stay on. Get going!

# CHAP2TER

# THE BIONIC BODY:
## What's the Matter
## with the One You've Got ?

**T**here is very little about exercise training that is metaphysical. With the recent massive popularity of sports and physical activity, it is not surprising that the uninformed should emerge with philosophical rather than physiological solutions to problems encountered in exercising. Make no mistake—any improvements that occur will be dictated by the laws of biology, chemistry, and physics, and not by some inner space you reach during training. Sports scientists are learning that exercise capacity improves at a predictable rate if you train at an optimal intensity. If you overload your body with a higher physiological load than you have in the past, you will improve. Work with your body as the engineer works with aluminum and steel. Support and reinforce weaknesses, and take advantage of strengths. If you apply the concepts necessary for improved physiological efficiency in a progressive and consistent manner, you will become physically fit. In fact, even an ordinary person with seemingly minimal physical abilities can reach high levels of skill and fitness. Concentrate on concrete factors. Systematically improve your metabolism, the strength and flexibility of your muscles, and the efficiency of your movements. Analyze your strengths and weaknesses and move in a positive direction. Your more philosophical friends may reach nirvana during your tennis match, but you'll be in the winner's circle.

## TIPPING THE BALANCE

The body always tries to seek a balance. The biologists call this balance homeostasis. It occurs at the level of least resistance. If your body is forced to perform heavy endurance exercise, then you will adjust, and the exercise will become easier. If, on the other hand, you are lazy and inactive, your body will adjust to a lower level of existence. You will not be capable of physically demanding tasks. Exercise training upsets your body balance. Your body is driven to improve its capacity; it adjusts— you become physically fit. However, once you have attained a higher level of body balance (i.e., physical fitness) you must continue to work out or you'll lose it. Your body perceives a period of inactivity as a new level of balance. It's easy to get out of shape. Physical fitness requires regular, consistent training. Irregular training could be dangerous and is most certainly painful and uncomfortable. You have to learn to enjoy the process of training, or there is no way that you'll stay on a lifetime program.

Your body reacts in a very specific way to different types of exercise. If you jog, the effects on your metabolism will be different than if you lift weights. Participation in a variety of sports and physical activities requires a diversified, well-rounded kind of physical fitness. Your program should be varied enough to make you quick and explosive for games such as tennis and racquetball, and yet provide enough endurance to allow you to enjoy a backpacking trip in the mountains. Total fitness requires adaptability. You must develop and stress your body in a number of different ways to be physically prepared for a variety of sports. To coin a phrase, "You are what you do." Your physical capacities are a direct result of the variety and intensity of your activites. You can't expect to leap tall buildings in a single bound if all you do is jog around the track.

We had the privilege of testing Bruce Jenner in our laboratory shortly before his gold medal decathlon performance at the Olympics. Although he was obviously a superbly conditioned athlete, we have studied other people with greater endurance or greater strength, greater muscle mass or more speed. Then why was Jenner hailed as one of the greatest athletes of all time? Because his physical abilities were well balanced. He was excellent in many categories. He was good in strength events, such as the discus and shot put, as well as in endurance events, such as the 1500-meter run. His fitness and skills were well rounded, and he exhibited his physical prowess at the highest level possible. He is probably the ultimate jock.

You are on a continuum with the decathlon athlete. It's certainly conceivable that Jenner could have been better in many of the events at the Olympics. You too can be better in the sports that you play. The essence of your improvements are similar to those of the greatest athlete in the world. In fact, you can expect to improve much more than the top sports people. While they require months or even years to make small improvements, you will make much larger gains because of your lower level of skill. You and the great athletes are subject to the same biological laws. You can compare yourself with the physically skilled because you are doing the same thing as they are. The essence is the same.

Like the decathlon athlete, the "Total Jock" fitness program demands balance. If you go overboard in one area, such as strength, you may bias your systems of metabolism to such an extent that it may be difficult to acquire the necessary endurance. The ability to run a 3½-hour marathon or bench press 300 pounds may not help you to hit a tennis ball any better, ski more gracefully, or sink a 20-foot jump shot. The successful jock has to develop the heart and lungs, the chemical processes within the cells, and the strength and flexibility of muscles, and you have to tie it all together with a razor-sharp nervous system that has been trained to react to a variety of situations rapidly and fluidly. Even if you are just beginning your program, try to work on several areas of your fitness. Do a few strength and flexibility exercises after running. Add a weekly game of tennis. It doesn't take that much time to develop a more well-rounded physical fitness.

Learn about yourself. Discover those aspects of your physiology that you can improve. Most of the great athletes whom I have known have been perfectionists. If they have weaknesses, they find out what they are and attempt to correct them. They get the most out of their practice sessions. If you spend your training time wisely, you will improve at a rapid rate in less time than you think. Become systematic. Your body is like a mound of clay—ready to be molded.

## THE BIOLOGICAL MACHINE

Top race drivers usually know as much about their cars as their mechanics do. They have a feel for when to nurse their machines around a curve and when to let it all hang out on the straightaways. They know how much fuel they will need to drive at a given speed. Their cars are highly predictable instruments. The racer learns the car's strengths and weaknesses. The most successful driver is often the one who knows exactly what to expect of his machine.

In many ways, your body is like a machine—a biological machine. A car burns gasoline that provides the energy to move. You utilize food that provides your body with energy to exercise. Just as the automobile requires a predictable amount of energy to drive 60 miles per hour, your body requires a predictable amount of energy to run a ten-minute mile. Unlike a machine, your body can adjust to stresses placed upon it. By regular application of the right amount of exercise stress, you can improve your fitness to very high levels. You can increase your exercise capacity rapidly if you realize that your body is like a precision machine.

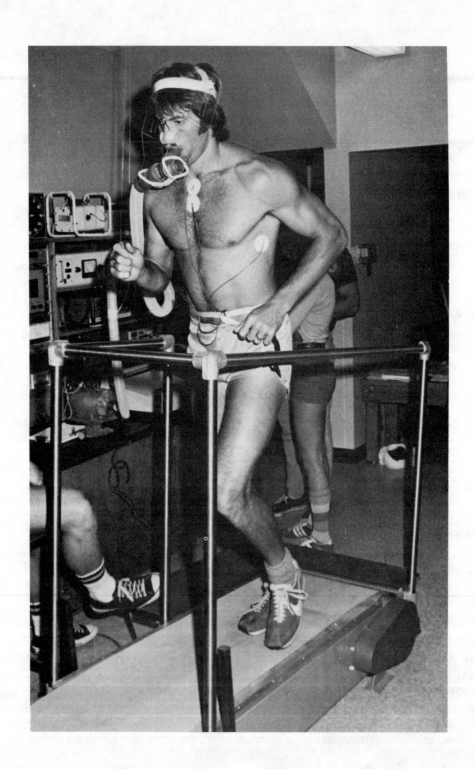

Your body breaks food down to provide energy, which is part of a complicated process called metabolism. You can express the amount of energy needed for a sport in terms of metabolism. For instance, your metabolic rate is increased more when you run than when you walk. Cross-country skiing requires a higher level of metabolism than playing golf. A given intensity of exercise will necessitate a predictable increase in the level of metabolism. In short, the harder you train, the more your metabolism increases. When you are working at a high metabolic rate, this means that you are transforming fuels so that they release energy very rapidly and in great quantities. In many sports, the efficiency of the metabolism determines whether you win or lose. Indeed, in sports like mountain climbing, if you don't have a high metabolic capacity you can't even participate.

Physical fitness implies the ability to increase your metabolic rate. Increasing the metabolic rate means that your body produces more energy so that you can do more exercise. The higher your metabolic rate, the more exercise you can perform. If you can run a six-minute mile, you can increase your metabolic rate more than a person who can run only a ten-minute mile. The faster runner uses fuel at a greater rate. There is a definite ceiling to the number of times you can increase your metabolic rate. A champion cross-country skier may be able to increase his metabolism 25 times, while a sedentary person who has had a recent heart attack may be able to increase it only five times. The ability to reach high levels of metabolism is determined by many factors, such as the fitness of cardiovascular system and the capacity of your muscle chemical systems. When you increase your metabolism, you increase the ability of your heart to pump blood and oxygen, and you increase the capacity of your muscle chemistry systems. The higher your metabolic capacity, the more exercise you can do. *High metabolic capacity and fitness are the same thing.*

I have chosen to express physical fitness as "max mets," i.e., the number of times the metabolism can be increased above rest. At rest you are at 1 met. In other words, 1 met is the same as your resting metabolism. When resting, your body requires a certain amount of energy to survive. This energy is equal to 1 met. When you exercise, your body must increase its metabolism so that you have enough energy. We express this increase in energy or metabolism in mets. So, when you

Bruce Jenner on the treadmill. Photo courtesy of Howard Lipin, *La Voz*, De Anza College newspaper.

increase your metabolism two times, you are exercising at 2 mets. When you increase this level ten times, you are working at 10 mets. The met cost of an activity tells you the number of times above rest you have to increase your metabolism. Your max mets tell you the number of times you are capable of increasing your metabolism above rest. The more you can increase your metabolism, the more exercise you can do. The higher your max mets, the more physically fit you are. I measure max mets in my laboratory with expensive computerized equipment. You can get a pretty good estimate of your max mets by performing some of the simple tests shown in Chapter 4. These tests invole walking, running, swimming, or biking as fast as you can over a certain distance. The faster you can cover the distance, the higher your max mets. Your max mets tell you your maximum energy level. They determine how long and how fast you can exercise.

The met cost of practically every sport or exercise has been carefully worked out by sports scientists over the past 35 years. Every sport has a met cost (see Chapter 4). Walking three miles in an hour has a cost of 3 mets. Running an eight-minute mile has a met cost of 14.5. Playing singles tennis has a met cost of between 4 and 9. By comparing your max mets with the met cost of a sport, you can see if you are in good enough shape to participate. The met cost of an exercise tells you its relative difficulty. Your max mets tells you your absolute maximum capacity.

As a "Total Jock" you will try to become involved in as many sports as possible. Your ability to participate in various activities is determined by the difficulty of the sport and your fitness. In Chapter 4, I have prepared an outline of the met cost of various sports and the minimum fitness in terms of max mets you will need to participate. To play any sport for a prolonged period of time (greater than 20 minutes), you should ideally have a max met capacity greater than 130–140 percent of the met cost of the sport you wish to play. For example, water skiing at a moderate intensity has a met cost of 5. You should have a minimum fitness level of 8 mets just to participate. Obviously, you can play a sport at different intensities. The harder you play at a sport, the more fit you have to be. When you become physically fit, you can perform these sports at 90 percent of your max mets. The goal of the "Total Jock" is to make you fit for sports. When you are fit, you can play harder for a longer period of time.

By using mets, you can get the most out of your biological machine. If you have a max mets of 15, and you go for a walk with an intensity of 3 mets, you know it's not improving your fitness. If your capacity is only 8 mets and someone asks you to climb a steep mountain, you will know that the met cost of the climb is above your present capacity. By increasing your max mets through training, you gradually increase your ability to participate in activities requiring high levels of metabolism. Training not only increases your max mets, but allows you to perform at a higher percentage of your maximum. When you get in shape, you will be able to ski and play tennis harder, and also longer, than ever before. The "Total Jock" program requires that you increase your max mets. The higher your mets, the more sports you can enjoy.

When using the met table, you must take into consideration the environment. The met costs of activities are similar at sea level, high altitude, and in hot and cold climates. However, your maximum capacity can be greatly affected by your surroundings. At 15,000 feet, mountain climbing has the same met cost as it does at 4,000 feet. The problem is that at that altitude, your maximum capacity could be cut by more than 25 percent. The relative difficulty of a sport is determined by the relationship of its met cost to your max mets. Your max mets are a lot less at 15,000 feet than at 6,000 feet, so climbing is a lot tougher at the higher elevation. High environmental temperature has a similar effect on performance. When your body becomes overheated, your max mets decrease, making a given sport more difficult.

## WHAT MAKES SAMMY RUN?

"What do you mean I'm not in top shape!" demanded Susan. "I play tennis at the club twice a week. With all of my housework, I probably get more exercise than a marathon runner."

The truth hurt Susan. She really thought she was in good shape because of the doubles games she played with her friends. But those two times a week were more like "once in a while." Her tennis game was really closer to "hit and go fetch." She was going through the motions. Susan is not unique. Many people have the illusion of fitness because they work with their hands or ski in the mountains a few times a year. Even though Susan was involved in a jock sport, she didn't have the major prerequisite for total sports enjoyment: a well-rounded physical fitness ready for many fun and exciting activities. Give her something a little more vigorous, like a backpacking trip or even a singles tennis match, and she would die on the vine.

The transition from rest to exercise is a lot like going from a peacetime to a wartime economy. Energy production is directed specifically at getting the job done. Your body's priorities are shifted toward pumping blood to your working muscles. All of your senses are geared to activity. Your body is seeking a higher level of balance.

Even before exercise actually begins, your body gets prepared. Your heart rate increases in anticipation. I have observed people so psyched up before their treadmill test that their heart rates exceed 150 beats per minute just thinking about running. Immediately before and during exercise, your body directs hormones and the nervous system toward facilitating the exercise.

When exercise begins, more blood must be pumped to the working muscles. The heart rate increases and continues to increase the harder you exercise. The heart also starts to pump more blood each time it beats (stroke volume). One of the biggest changes that happens from training is to increase the amount of blood ejected from your heart every time it beats. This saves a lot of work for the heart. Now your heart doesn't have to beat as often—it can pump the same amount of blood with a lower heart rate.

The harder you exercise, the more blood your heart must pump. Your muscles must get oxygen or they can't go on. There is a definite ceiling to the amount of blood your heart can pump. The more blood your heart pumps, the more exercise you can do. Training improves your heart's ability to pump. In fact, a physically fit person's heart may be able to pump twice as much blood as an unfit one.

Moving blood from inactive tissues to working muscles is extremely important in maintaining body balance during exercise. When you are out of shape, inefficiency in redistributing blood to your working muscles may contribute to fatigue. Moving blood to your exercising muscles is quite a job for your body. At rest your muscles receive about 15 percent of your total blood volume. During heavy exercise, as much as 85 percent of your blood flow must be transferred to your working tissues. You've got to open up blood vessels where they are needed, and close them where they aren't needed. Exercise training makes it a lot easier to get the blood to your muscles.

Fitness requires that you regularly push your body harder than before. You have to force your heart to pump more blood. You have to

Sports like archery require consistency.

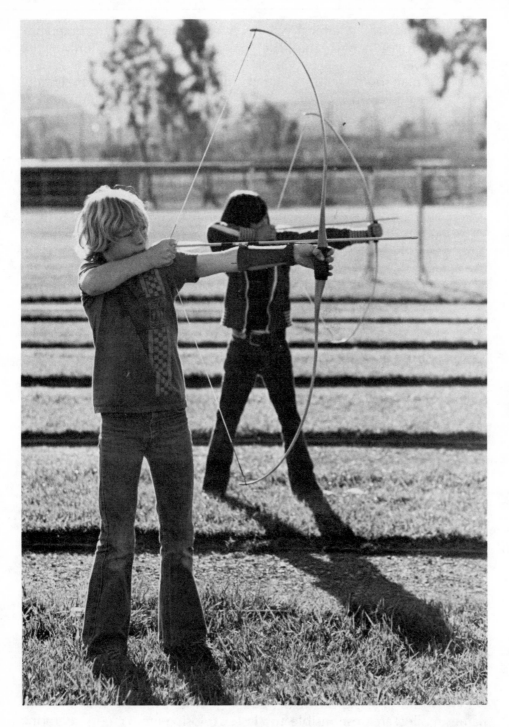

The Bionic Body    **35**

force your muscles' chemical systems to reach higher levels of metabolism. The process is enjoyable; the goal is a type of freedom only a jock can describe.

To play sports well, you need a fit cardiovascular system. Endurance is needed even in sports like bowling where the movements last only a few seconds. Sports like bowling, golf, or archery require consistency. Consistency drops off tremendously when you are fatigued. Fatigue may make you change that club position enough to miss an important shot. Exercise scientists have found that fatigue decreases your ability to learn sports skills. Improving your endurance will increase your effective practice time. Practicing when you are tired is wasted time. When you are exhausted, you can develop bad habits that you may never get rid of. Get in shape, and you increase your effective practice time. Make those practice sessions count.

## FAST AND FURIOUS

The "Total Jock" can do a lot more than run in a straight line for 20 minutes. You must be prepared for many sports: sports that require endurance; sports that require power and speed; and sports that require skill. More work is needed, but what difference does that make? The work is fun. A well-planned, systematic program will help you develop the well-rounded fitness needed for the sporting life.

Scientists have recently discovered that your body experiences different effects from endurance and high intensity exercise. In fact, you use different muscle cells within the same large tissue muscle to perform movements gently or forcefully. The effects of distance running are different from the effects of playing racquetball or sprinting. There is a specificity of training. The met cost of an activity doesn't completely reveal its demands on your body. Powder skiing, though demanding tremendous endurance, also requires shock-absorber knees and the ability to exert a lot of energy in a short period of time. To make your body ready for sports, you have to consider the physical demands. Few sports require only endurance, only strength, or only speed. Fitness for sports requires a combination of many types of physical fitness. The jock not only has a heart that can pump effectively, but a body that's flexible, strong, and skilled.

Your muscles are composed of two primary types of fibers: fast twitch (white) and slow twitch (red). Fast twitch muscle fibers, as the name implies, are responsible for fast, explosive movements requiring

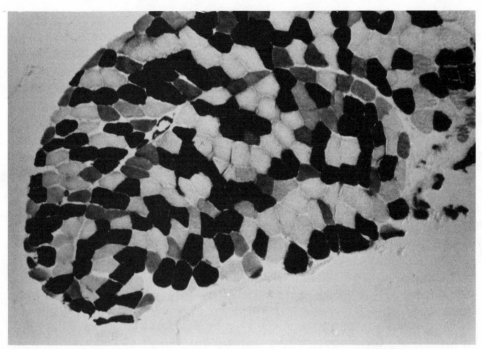

Human muscle: dark fibers are slow twitch; light fibers are two types of fast twitch. Photo courtesy of D. Costill, Human Performance Laboratory, Ball State University, Muncie, Indiana.

power. When you sprint or play racquetball or tennis, your fast twitch muscle fibers are doing much of the work. Slow twitch fibers are used for endurance exercise, such as jogging. You can have more of one type of fiber than another in a muscle group. If you have a predominance of fast twitch fibers in your legs, then you are likely to be a good sprinter. If you have more red fibers, you will have better endurance. Studies by sports scientists have shown that the top endurance athletes have a predominance of slow twitch fibers and top strength athletes have more fast twitch fibers. Good examples of fast and slow twitch muscles can be seen at the dinner table. Ducks, who fly great distances and have tremendous endurance, are predominantly dark meat (slow twitch). Grouse, who don't have great endurance but fly like lightning, are primarily white meat (fast twitch). Present scientific evidence suggests that you are born with a fixed percentage of fast twitch or slow twitch muscle. Most people have similar percentages of each fiber type. Your program should include sports and exercises that use both types of fibers.

There are distinct differences between the fibers in structure, function, and the way fuel is transformed to energy for exercise. Slow twitch fibers depend upon oxygen and fuels delivered by the blood.

They have a large blood supply. Slow twitch fibers have numerous small energy centers called mitochondria that are responsible for consuming oxygen and providing energy for exercise. Fats as well as carbohydrates are an extremely important source of fuel for these fibers. Slow twitch fibers have a lot of endurance; they release energy slowly for long periods but aren't very strong.

Fast twitch fibers are faster, larger, stronger, but fatigue faster. Their main fuel is a complex sugar called glycogen. These fibers need less oxygen and contain fewer energy centers (mitochondria). The blood supply is less; they recover from fatigue more slowly.

Endurance, speed, and power exercises exert different effects on your body. Endurance exercise develops your heart's ability to pump blood and the ability of your muscles to burn fats and consume oxygen. Endurance training is aimed at allowing your metabolism to operate for a long time. It is not unusual for a distance runner to cover 150 miles per week or for a swimmer to put in 15,000 meters in a workout. High-intensity exercise develops your ability to produce energy at a very fast rate. You develop the ability of your muscles to contract faster and with more power. Fast-acting muscle enzymes needed for optimum speed and power are developed in high-intensity training.

Total fitness requires many types of training because the effects of exercise are so specific. When you run or swim long distances or go on a ten-mile hike in the mountains, you train your slow twitch fibers. All this endurance training does little to improve the performance of your fast twitch fibers. If you run four miles a day and don't ever do any sprint training, you will never increase your speed for games like tennis or handball. I don't care how much weight you lift, you're not going to develop cardiovascular endurance unless you perform regular endurance exercise. Your body will improve in the areas that it is trained. Sprint training improves the performance of your fast twitch fibers, and endurance training improves the performance of your slow twitch fibers. Your training program should get you ready for many sports. When you play tennis, ski, or surf, you need strength, power, and endurance. Get your body ready for a lot of activities. Prepare yourself for many sports. Develop a well-rounded physical fitness.

## BORN OR MADE

Mac Wilkins, Olympic gold medal winner in the discus, picked up the hammer in a meet in Europe and threw over 200 feet. Wilkins' throw made him one of the top hammer throwers in the United States. This wouldn't have surprised anyone—except that he had thrown hammer only a few times before. We all know many people who are naturally good at sports. These people are sometimes called natural athletes. Why is it that people like Wilkins can perform well in so many activities, while the rest of us have to work so hard for much more modest gains?

To a large extent you are born with your physical abilities. Most of us couldn't run a four-minute mile if we trained from now until doomsday. Does this mean that you are doomed to mediocrity if you didn't happen to choose the right parents? No! Although there is a ceiling to your ultimate physical capacity, you probably won't begin to scratch the surface. You have a tremendous capacity for improvement. With the right training program and enough self-confidence, you can make great improvements in your skill and fitness. You must learn to make the best of what you have. You can make your movement more efficient, increase your endurance, and become stronger. Genetics may keep you from an Olympic gold medal, but hard work and consistent training can bring you up to a respectable level of performance, even if you are just beginning.

Exercise scientists from the Washington University School of Medicine in St. Louis have recently demonstrated that it is possible to develop endurance capacity almost 50 percent in as little as ten weeks. Their exercise program involved exhaustive levels of training, five days a week. Although the daily training time was less than an hour, previously out-of-shape people developed the endurance capacity of trained athletes. Rapid gains were made because the training loads were increased systematically. Whenever improvements were made, the exercise intensity was increased: The workout got harder. This type of program is not very practical for the average person; it is certainly not very enjoyable. If you were to try exercising at this level on a regular basis, you might easily become injured. I think, though, that this study illustrates the great capacity of the human machine to improve. Maybe you won't improve 50 percent in ten weeks, but you may improve 5 percent. That 5 percent may be the difference between victory and defeat or, more importantly, whether you have fun or not.

You must believe in yourself and in your ability to improve. If it's not in your head, the idea will never be transmitted to the rest of your body. Don't let your head convince you that you can't become a jock. Your body is ready. Do something with it. When Vince Lombardi first took over as coach of the Green Bay Packers, the players were the whipping boys of the National Football League. He transformed them

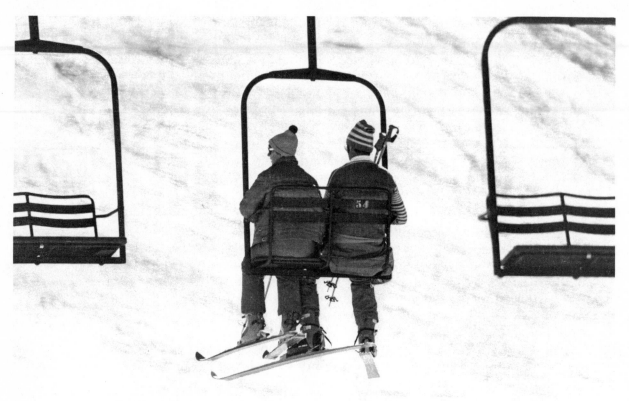

Rest on the chair

from losers to perennial winners. They were the same players, but he molded them into a precision instrument. When you believe that you can take your body and make it do what you want, you will improve. Overload your body consistently, and you can overcome not having Olympic champions as parents. And you can make these improvements without working as hard as a pro football player.

Lombardi and other great coaches have been successful because they never left anything to chance. They never became complacent. They felt no athlete was ever too good to improve. Structure your program for excellence. In every game, no matter what the arena, there is a winner and a loser. You may as well pick the winning side. Even if winning for you is simply playing well and having fun, pick the winning side. Your body can meet the vast majority of your expectations if you push yourself in the right direction.

# WHY YOU GET TIRED

"I don't understand it," complained Betty, "I can't seem to make it through a whole day of skiing without feeling exhausted. I've always considered myself active. I jog a couple of times a week—there must be something wrong with me."

I suggested to Betty that she see her physician for a medical exam. The results indicated she was in good health. She then underwent a series of tests in my laboratory. We first weighed her under water to measure her body fat and muscle mass. The results showed her to be 31 percent fat, well over the ideal maximum of 25 percent. We tested her on the treadmill to measure her oxygen consumption, electrocardiogram, and blood pressure. She achieved a fitness level of 10 mets. Her EKG indicated that her heart was functioning normally. We then gave her a complete battery of strength and flexibility tests. Her scores were about 30 percent less than the desirable levels required for skiing.

Betty is typical of a lot of people. She can't enjoy strenuous sports because of fatigue. Although I wouldn't call her a physical wreck, she just didn't have the fitness required to enjoy such a demanding sport as skiing. She was carrying around too much fat. Those extra pounds were making her work harder, and they made balancing on skis more difficult. Her fitness level of 10 mets was barely adequate to meet the demands of skiing even at a low intensity. Her lack of strength and flexibility not only contributed to her fatigue but made her more susceptible to serious injury. Betty got tired because her body was not trained to meet the energy demands of skiing. She was deficient in many areas of fitness, not just endurance. I suggested a program that would develop a well-rounded metabolism. Her exercise training was designed to meet the energy demands of many sports.

The energy requirements of sports have to be met or you won't be able to continue for very long. The fitness requirements of sports are considerably more varied than those of most conditioning exercises. Jogging, for example, improves endurance, but does little to develop strength, speed, or power. When you play sports like tennis, you need more than stamina. You need power, speed, and agility. If you lack any component of fitness required for a sport, you will tire easily. That's why the "Total Jock" needs a well-rounded fitness program. Betty probably would have become tired skiing even with a higher endurance capacity. Her poor muscle strength would have caused her to fatigue rapidly.

For high-intensity sports, you must not only produce energy in great quantities, you must produce it rapidly. It's the rate that counts. Often a step is all that separates the person who makes a shot from the person who doesn't. If you're consistently a stride away because of lack of speed, it doesn't matter how much stamina you have. All you have developed from your jogging program is the endurance to lose all day. Remember, training is specific. If you are going to play at high intensities,.you have to train that way. You have to mold your metabolism to perform the way you want it to.

Physiologically, the causes of fatigue are difficult to pin down. Fatigue appears to be related to a variety of factors, depending upon the type of sport or exercise. Some apparently obvious causes really have little to do with the fatigue process. Breathing difficulties, for example, are universally blamed for early tiring during exercise. Unless you have a lung disease, such as emphysema or asthma, or you are exercising at high altitude, breathing has little to do with your symptoms.

In endurance work, your heart's ability to pump blood (cardiac output) is a leading limiting factor. Many sensations commonly associated with fatigue, such as a weakening in the legs and a general feeling of exhaustion, can be directly linked to the ability of your heart to pump enough blood through your muscles. The best way to improve your heart's ability to pump blood is to include endurance exercise as part of your program. Probably more than any other factor, the capacity of your heart controls when you are going to get tired. In fact, your heart's pumping ability will often determine if you are going to enjoy a sport. If an activity is beyond the capacity of your metabolism, you're not going to enjoy it very much.

Another important source of fatigue in both endurance and high-intensity exercise is the depletion of fuel sources within your muscles. Sugars or carbohydrates are the major source of fuel for muscular work of high intensity. Even in endurance exercise, where the burning of fats is more significant, the carbohydrate stores in your muscles determine how long you can go on. When your muscles' sugar stores (glycogen) run out, you have hit the endurance wall. Exercise becomes difficult. At that point you had better hope the game gets rained out.

Staleness, a condition encountered by most serious jocks at one time or another, is when your performances deteriorate in spite of heavy training. You may become stale when you jog too many miles in a week or play too many hours of tennis. This condition may be caused by the depletion of sugar stores in your muscle  and liver. Rest and increasing the carbohydrate content of your diet are the only things that will pull you out of it.

If you try to increase your training when you are stale, you will feel worse instead of better. A runner from our college track team came to the laboratory for advice because his performances were deteriorating during the track season. Every time he ran a bad race he would train harder. The result: a slower time the next week. He was also on a low-carbohydrate, high-protein diet to lose weight, which didn't help matters much. He was suffering from the classic symptoms of glycogen depletion (low sugar in muscles and liver). I advised him to take five days off and to increase the carbohydrate content of his diet. The result was his best performance of the year, and he broke out of the staleness that was plaguing him.

Maintaining your muscle and liver sugar stores is one thing you can do to improve your performance and help stave off fatigue. By combining a high-performance diet with the right combination of rest and exercise, you will be ready for top performance.

In high-intensity exercise, such as sprinting, several factors may be significant in limiting performance. In a sense the fatigue process is a competition between the energy supply and demand of your metabolism. You can exercise effectively only as long as you have an adequate energy supply. One sign that your metabolism is losing the battle is the accumulation of acid. If the oxygen supply to your muscles is inadequate, or if you are exercising hard and using those fast twitch muscles, glycogen breaks down to lactic acid in your muscles. You continually produce substances such as lactic acid. Usually this is not a problem, because your muscles use it or give it up to the cleansing blood flow as fast as it is produced. When the lactic acid levels get very high, however, as in high-intensity exercise, this may cause enough pain to make you quit or it may interfere with chemical reactions within your muscles that are necessary for continuing exercise.

Dr. George Brooks, a leading exercise biochemist from the University of California, has found that muscle temperatures get very high during heavy exercise. This may produce a condition where oxygen is being consumed, but less energy is available for exercise. The causes of fatigue during heavy exercise are not completely understood and are certainly controversial. On a practical level, the best thing you can do is prepare your body for the demands of exercise. "Total Jock" sports require endurance, speed, strength, flexibility, and agility. Your fitness program should reflect these demands. You have to have a well-rounded program.

# AND EXERCISE WON'T ROT YOUR TEETH

Improved health is a natural result of the "Total Jock" program. Although I don't think that prevention of heart disease should be your primary reason for exercising, the jock lifestyle may help you avoid heart problems.

There is ample evidence that regular physical exercise will make you feel better and significantly reduce your risk of heart attack. I have to agree with Dr. P.O. Astrand of Sweden, a leading exercise physiologist, who said, "I'm not going to wait a hundred years for scientists to prove conclusively that exercise is good for you. I am going to lead an active life now. I think if you are not going to exercise, you should see a doctor to determine if you can withstand a sedentary existence."

For years, scientists have tried to establish a link between physical activity and reduced risk of heart disease. John Morris, a British researcher, studied people in several active and sedentary occupations. He compared bus drivers (sedentary) and conductors (active), postal clerks (sedentary) and postmen (active), and telegraphers (active) and telephone operators (sedentary). In all cases the active occupations had lower levels of heart disease. Doctors Pomeroy and White studied 355 Harvard football players of 1901–1939 and investigated the cause of death of 87 who died. None of the former players who continued to exercise showed evidence of heart disease, while 25 of the less active men suffered heart attacks.

Numerous other studies have been conducted. Some seemed to link exercise with a decreased risk, while other studies could show no relationship. The problem with all of these investigations is the inability of the scientists to quantify the fitness levels. For example, even though mail deliverers are more active than postal clerks, the activity level of both groups is really pretty low. In my laboratory I have not found people in active occupations to be any more fit than people employed in sedentary jobs. Unless they regularly stressed their body above 50 percent of their max mets (maximum capacity), they were not training on the job to become physically fit.

Dr. Ken Cooper evaluated nearly 3,000 men at the Aerobics Center in Dallas. He was able to demonstrate a direct link between physical fitness and a lower risk of heart disease. Cooper found that people with higher fitness capacities (max mets) had lower resting heart rates, body weight, body fat, blood fats (cholesterol and triglycerides), blood glucose, and blood pressure. Cooper used precise methods to determine physical fitness and body fat. His data show that physical exercise is a lot more important in preventing heart attack than most health experts have suspected.

The relationship of cholesterol and heart disease has been a subject of controversy for many years. Statistically there is a relationship between the incidence of heart disease and cholesterol levels in the blood. However, studies in which subjects lowered cholesterol through diet were unable to show any beneficial effect in lessening the incidence of heart disease. Scientists have recently demonstrated a relationship between substances called lipoproteins and cardiovascular disease. There are three primary types of lipoproteins: very low-density lipoproteins (VLDL), low-density lipoproteins (LDL), and high-density lipoproteins (HDL). Increased concentrations of the low-density faction, LDL, is associated with an increased development of hardening of the arteries. HDL, however, seems to actually retard the development of coronary artery disease. It is better to have more high-density lipoprotein. Researchers at the Stanford Heart Disease Prevention Center have shown that physical exercise reduces the low-density lipoproteins, LDL, while raising the level of high-density lipoproteins. For the first time physical exercise has been linked to the prevention of a condition directly involved in the development of coronary artery disease.

Emotional stress is another factor identified with increased risk of heart disease. Everyone seems to be stressed about stress in our society. Numerous books are written about stress; countless seminars are conducted about stress; and television presents situation comedies about stress. Stress is a national obsession. We are urged to avoid stressful situations. We are told not to drive in the fast lane and not to jump from the long line to the short line. We are told not to jog or play singles tennis because this makes us stressful. We are told not to compete.

Remember, stress is what urges you on to excellence. It's not the stress that is dangerous, but the way you cope with stress. In many societies people are under a lot of stress but don't get heart attacks. What makes you think the stresses you endure are any greater than those of certain African societies? They're stressed about things like food and clothing. Their survival stress is just as pressing as the stress you feel from plummeting stock prices or from lack of money to purchase a fancy new car. Although many factors are involved, active societies have lower levels of heart disease than sedentary societies. In the United States since 1973 there has been a marked decrease in the heart attack rate among business executives. Business personnel are under the same amount of stress that they've always been under. The difference is that they've become aware of the beneficial effect of physical activity and of reducing the fat content of their diets.

The effects of exercise on stress can be measured. In stressful situations, such as when someone cuts you off on the freeway, you secrete hormones called catacholamines. Adrenalin is an example of a catacholamine. These hormones overload your cardiovascular system and speed up the process of hardening of the arteries. Exercise training reduces the cardiovascular response of catacholamine during stress. When you are involved in an exercise program, stress has less effect on your body. You get this protection against stress even if you are a stressful jogger or the kind of tennis player who breaks your racquet over the net post when you lose.

Is exercise safe? Let's just say it's more dangerous to be sedentary than to exercise. Dr. Jockl of the University of Tennessee has studied many cases of deaths during exercise. He was unable to identify any cases where death occurred in people with healthy hearts. If you have heart disease, exercise without supervision can be potentially dangerous. I would suggest that before you begin a serious program that you (1) get a physical exam, (2) have an electrocardiogram taken on a bicycle or treadmill, and (3) have a systematic plan for improvement. The safey of jogging has been carefully documented at the Aerobics Center in Dallas. There have been only a few mishaps during thousands of miles of training. You are in just as much danger exercising as of being struck by lightning or hit by a falling tree.

You will probably be more susceptible to aches and pains on the "Total Jock" exercise program than jogging or swimming slowly. If you aren't in very good shape now, I have outlined a development program to prepare you for more rigorous training. If you start out slowly and sensibly, you won't get injured. You have to learn to build upon what you have. You have a lot of time to become involved in the process of an active life.

## INSTANT REPLAY

1. Your body reacts to the stresses placed upon it. To improve your physical fitness you must consistently increase the severity of your workouts.
2. Training is specific. Your training programs should be varied to provide endurance, strength, flexibility, speed, and skill.
3. Mets are the multiple of the resting metabolic rate. Mets can be used to quantify the energy cost of a sport (met cost). Your max mets is the number of times you can increase your metabolism above rest. Max mets is a measure of your physical fitness. By comparing your max mets with the met cost of a sport, you can determine if you're in shape.
4. When you go from rest to exercise, your blood is shunted to the working muscles; your heart rate and the amount of blood pumped by the heart increase. Training increases the amount of blood your heart can pump and the efficiency of the blood distribution.
5. Training increases the efficiency of the chemical systems within your muscles.
6. Your muscles contain two primary types of fibers: fast twitch and slow twitch. Fast twitch fibers enable you to perform movements rapidly with great force. Slow twitch fibers enable you to perform exercises longer.
7. Carbohydrates are the major fuel for high-intensity exercise. It's important to have an adequate supply of carbohydrates in your diet.
8. Exercise may reduce your chances of getting heart disease.

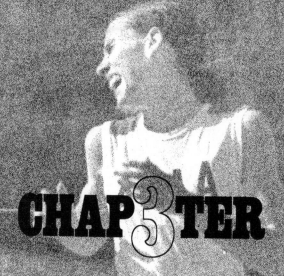

# CHAP3TER

# NO PAIN-NO GAIN:
# The Principles of Training

Exercise and sports have always been surrounded by myth and tradition. Practices that started out as the whim of some coach or athlete often became institutionalized and were passed down from one generation to the next. Some of these are undoubtedly correct, having stood the test of time as solid training principles. The overload principle, the maxim that you must subject your body to increasing exercise loads to improve your fitness, is a time-honored concept with origins in ancient Greece. Milo of Crote, a top wrestler of the time, is said to have hoisted a young calf upon his shoulders and walked around with it. He did this every day. As the calf grew to maturity, Milo increased his strength. Milo was unbeatable after his unusual training program. He laid the foundation for modern weight training methods.

There are equally old concepts that have not stood the test of scientific scrutiny. Ancient warriors believed that by eating meat, especially raw meat, they could increase their strength and muscle mass. These warriors also believed that by eating the heart of a courageous enemy they would become braver and fiercer in battle. To this day, athletes still believe increased protein will make them stronger. I have no information on how many of them also eat the hearts of their competitors. Recent studies of the protein requirements of trained men and women show that their protein needs are not any greater than those of sedentary people (about 1 gram per kilogram body weight).

On any given day you are deluged with sales pitches for exercise gadgets that promise instant fitness in only a few minutes a day. If you learn the basic principles of training, you can ferret out the frauds. You will be able to progress at the fastest possible rate with the least amount of pain and discomfort. In this chapter I will attempt to answer some of the commonly asked questions about sports and exercise training.

# TRAINING PRINCIPLES
## What is the Overload Principle?

The overload principle is the basis of any training program. It states that you must subject your body to increasing exercise intensities to experience any improvement of fitness. This principle depends upon the tendency of your body to adjust to physical stress. Endurance, speed, strength, flexibility, and perhaps even skill level depend upon the overload principle for improvement.

This principle, if applied consistently and over a prolonged period of time, will result in greatly improved fitness in many areas of performance. For example, if you consistently try to run a little faster and a little further, your endurance will increase. Lifting a little more weight each week will make you stronger. You will have your ups and downs. Sometimes you will go out on the track with the intention of breaking your personal record. The result may be that you run 30 seconds slower than you did a month ago. Setbacks are a part of training. But, if you continue to apply the overload principle consistently, you will improve.

The extent of your improvement will be determined by your genetic ceiling, the time you spend training, and your ultimate level of aspiration. The endurance of a marathon runner is not necessary. Although endurance exercise is an important part of your program, you need time for sports and exercises to develop your strength, flexibility, and speed. After you reach an optimal level of fitness, your program will center around maintenance of condition. Sports and games will take center ring. After you have become fit, you can really experience the active way of life.


## How Much Training Time Do I Need to Get Into Shape?

Almost anyone can reach a reasonable degree of fitness in six to eight months. Fitness involves more than endurance, so a well-rounded type of physical fitness may take you quite some time. Because you are shooting for all-around capacity, you will not necessarily develop the endurance of a distance runner or the strength of a weight lifter.

The overload principle is the principle of any training program—you have to subject your body to increasing exercise intensities to experience any improvement in fitness.

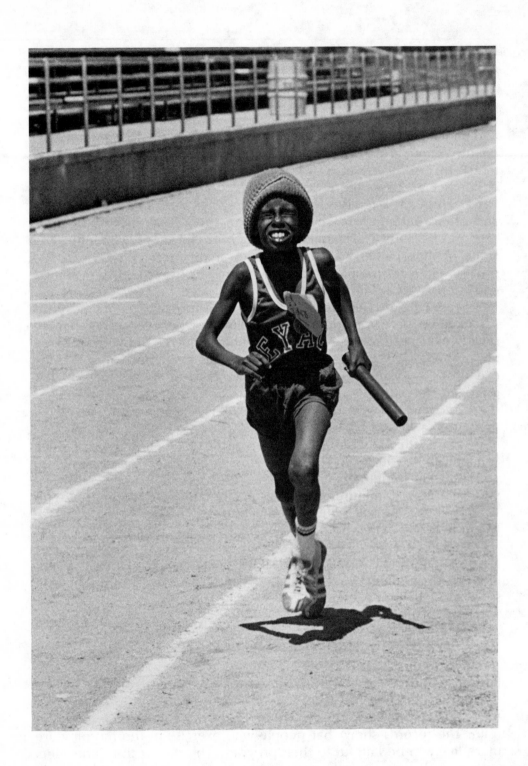

However, you can reach respectable levels in many areas of performance.

You have to have a minimum level of endurance for total sports participation. Count on training continuously above 60 percent of your maximum capacity for at least 20 minutes, three to five times per week. Endurance exercises such as jogging, swimming, cycling, or cross-country skiing are a must for developing your metabolic capacity (max mets). In fact, if you have a limited amount of time for training, the endurance exercises should come first.

Flexibility exercises should be a regular part of your day. Before and after running, you should perform the "Total Jock" stretching exercises (Chapter 7). Flexibility training will help you prevent injury and some of those aches and pains that invariably accompany a training program. In many people, regular stretching will help to prevent chronic conditions such as low back pain.

Speed exercises are important for performance of many sports (Chapter 5). There is an increased risk of injury whenever you train more rapidly. You can minimize the danger of high-speed training by warming up properly and by performing an adequate amount of stretching exercises. Too much speed work will tend to deplete your muscles' glycogen stores (fuel) and make exercise performance more difficult. I don't recommend you do high-speed exercises any more frequently than twice a week.

Strength exercises should be practiced at least twice a week (Chapter 6). If you try to strength train any less than that you will find your isolated strength exercise sessions result in muscle soreness. Even if you train only 15 minutes a session on strength, you can improve this type of fitness. To reach high levels of strength, however, you will have to put in at least three hours a week and probably much more.

The more time you have to put in on exercises the better. As long as you're enjoying yourself, spend all the time you want. Fun is the most important ingredient of your program. If you're having fun, you haven't spent too much time.

## What's the Best Time of Day to Train?

Basically, individual preference dictates the time of day you train. At the Aerobic Center in Dallas, where there is a computer terminal outside of the locker room, accurate records are kept on the times their members train. The records show that people who exercise in the morning are more likely to be faithful to their program. The staff at the Center feel the answer lies in human nature. If exercise is the first thing you do in the morning, you're likely to get it done. After work or dinner, when you're tired or full, you can think of a thousand reasons to take it easy.

I would advise against strenuous exercise in the middle of the day during the hot days of summer. Dehydration and thermal distress are a problem for many people. The heat can be particularly dangerous if you are not in good physical condition.

## What is Specificity of Training?

The principle of specificity of training provides that your physical preparation should closely approximate the sport. This principle is extremely important in helping you minimize wasted time on the playing field. When strengthening muscles for a sport, work on the ones used. If you're training to paddle a canoe, it doesn't do you very much good to do leg-strengthening exercises. If you're going to play handball, more than distance running is needed to prepare you physically. Practice for the sports you're going to do. Because you want to do many sports, you must prepare yourself in many ways.

The more closely you can approximate the movement, the more productive your program will be. When you are practicing a skill, try to execute it at the same speed that is required in the sport. Even though breaking a movement down into parts may be helpful, you have to perform it at a realistic speed.

Fatigue is an important consideration in learning a skill. When you are exhausted, you practice a skill differently than when you're fresh. Practicing when you are overly tired is not efficient use of training time.

Strength training particularly should be practiced with specificity in mind. Train those muscles that are used in a motion. Ideally, you should overload your muscles in the same movement and at the same speed required in the sport.

If your program is consistent with the principle of specificity, you will save time and improve at the fastest rate. Remember, train the way you hope to perform. If you have to move fast, train fast.

## HOW CAN I PREVENT INJURY?

You can prevent injury primarily by being in top physical condition. High-intensity sports requiring rapid changes of direction (tennis, rac-

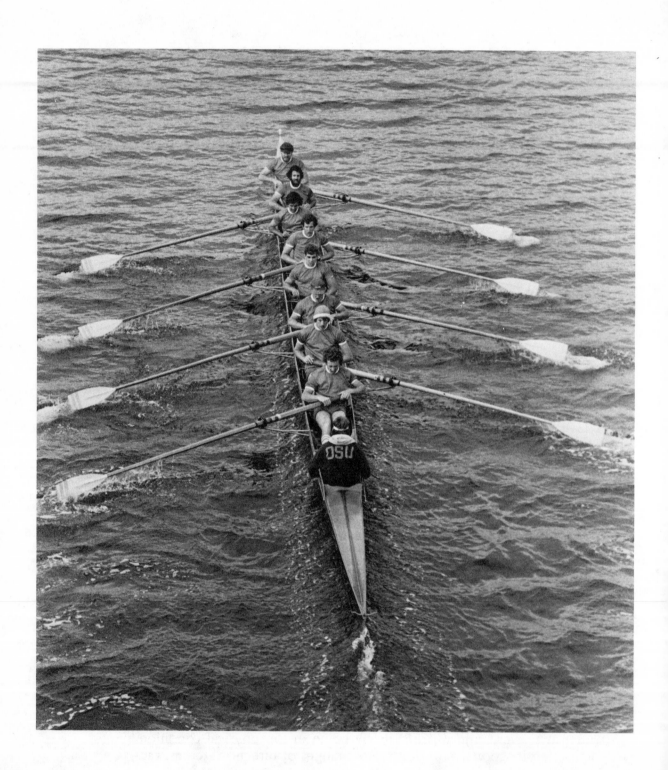

quetball, basketball) or resistance to tremendous external forces (skiing, surfing, or water skiing) often have increased risk of injury. Making sure the muscles supporting your joints are strong and flexible will minimize the possibility of your getting hurt.

Start slowly. Many injuries are brought on by training too hard, too soon. I'm always very concerned when I run into an out-of-shape, middle-aged man who was an athlete in school. He may be suffering from the "Old Pro Syndrome." These men sometimes think they can do the same things they did in their 20's. A 25-second 220-yard dash may be no problem for a 20-year-old, but when a 45-year-old tries it his hamstrings may "roll up like a scroll." If you start slowly and build, you will prevent shin splints, sore feet, and painful knees.

Warm-up is very important. Warm-up involves preliminary exercises to prepare your body for exercise. The warm-up helps to deliver blood to your muscles and facilitate their elastic properties. The slightly elevated muscle temperature caused by the warm-up helps the muscles convert fuels to energy faster and more efficiently. Researchers from UCLA have found that your heart needs a warm-up as well: People with healthy hearts developed abnormalities in the electrocardiogram when they did sprint running without warm-up.

Flexibility exercises have resulted in significant reduction of injuries on several professional football teams. Many muscle and joint injuries result from body parts being forced beyond their range of motion capacity. By increasing this capacity, you diminish the risk of injury. In Chapter 7, I will present many useful exercises to increase your flexibility and minimize the chances of injury.

Running surfaces are also critical. I recommend that you run on grass or other soft surfaces. You want to minimize the jarring you get from running. If you can't avoid pavement, then get shoes designed for hard surfaces.

I can't stress the importance of fitness enough. The unfit fatigue rapidly. The tired jock is the one who is injured easily.

## HOW CAN I DETERMINE MY MAX METS?

Your max mets tell the number of times you can increase your metabolism above rest (1 met = 3.5 milliliters of oxygen consumed per kilogram

Rowing requires strength and endurance.

body weight). In the laboratory, I measure max mets on a treadmill or stationary bicycle with expensive gas analysis equipment and a computer. Exercise scientists have determined the energy costs of many activities. By knowing the intensity of walking, running, swimming, or bicycling, it's easy to calculate the met cost. In Chapter 4, I've outlined simple tests to determine your max mets. These tests are one- and three-mile walks; 1½-mile run; 400-yard swim; and three-mile bicycle ride. The faster you complete each of these tests, the higher your max mets for that activity. Simple tables will allow you to determine your max mets from your time.

Remember, your max mets determine the sports you can participate in. Mets tell you the energy requirement of a sport, and your max mets tell you your maximum energy capacity. If you have a high max mets, you can participate in sports requiring a lot of energy. With high max mets, you protect yourself from fatigue and injury.

## CAN I USE HEART RATE TO DETERMINE MY EXERCISE INTENSITY?

Heart rate is the most practical method of controlling the intensity of your exercise. Under ordinary circumstances at sea level and a comfortable temperature, your heart rate will give you an idea of the metabolic level you're working at. By performing your endurance exercises between 70 and 85 percent of your maximum heart rate (target heart rate), you will be training at an adequate intensity to improve your fitness. You'll get a ball-park estimate of your maximum heart rate by subtracting your age from 220. So, if you're 30 years old, your predicted maximum heart rate should be about 190 beats per minute (220 – 30 = 190). Your target heart rate is the level of exercise that will result in a training effect. Approximate target heart rates are as follows:

| Age | Target Heart Rate |
|---|---|
| 20 | 160–170 |
| 30 | 154–160 |
| 40 | 147–153 |
| 50 | 140–145 |
| 60 | 133–138 |

These values assume your maximum heart rate to be the average for your age. I've seen people in their 60's with maximum heart rates over 200 beats per minute and people in their 20's with maximum rates less than 160.

The best way to determine your maximum heart rate is during a treadmill test under the supervision of trained personnel. To determine if you've been exercising at your target heart rate, take your pulse for ten seconds immediately after exercise. Multiply this value by six. The following table gives some examples:

| Ten-Second Heart Rate | One-Minute Heart Rate |
|:---:|:---:|
| 15 | 90 |
| 20 | 120 |
| 25 | 150 |
| 30 | 180 |

Obviously a mistake of a few beats can make quite a difference. Count the first pulse you feel as zero. Count "zero, one, two, three," and so forth. It's very important to take your pulse immediately after exercise. If you wait 30 seconds, your heart rate will decrease. The heart rate you get as soon as you stop is the same one you've been training at.

The best way to measure your pulse is by placing your fingers directly over your heart or wrist. The neck or carotid pulse, which many people use to measure heart rate, will sometimes be slightly lower because palpating that site will stimulate your vagus nerve, which slows down your heart rate. In addition, taking the pulse at the neck may cut the supply of blood to your brain if you press too hard.

Heart rate is useful in determining training levels only for continuous rhythmic endurance exercises such as running, cycling, and swimming. Heart rate is deceiving for intermittent activities such as tennis, skiing, and racquetball. Even though levels may reach maximum for short periods, they drop dramatically during other periods. Measuring your heart rate while performing strength exercises, such as weight training, is essentially useless. Exercises involving straining causes the heart rate and blood pressure to rise disproportionately to the metabolism. Use heart rate as a conditioning index only for endurance exercise. You can increase your heart rate by sitting in your car during rush hour, watching scary movies, or looking at members of the opposite sex—but they're not endurance exercises.

The heart rate can be very useful for monitoring the correct exercise levels at high altitudes or in the heat. For example, your capacity decreases about 3 percent for every 1,000 feet above 6,000 feet. Walking four miles per hour at 10,000 feet still costs about 4 mets, but your capacity is less. A workout you can do easily at sea level will be more difficult at altitude. If you run a ten-minute mile at a heart rate of 150 beats per minute at sea level, the rate for the same workout will be higher at altitude. The met cost of the run is the same, but your max mets are lower.

Using your target heart rate will help you exercise at a comfortable rate while continuing to improve. Your pulse rate is your built-in performance indicator. Today your pulse may be 165 while running a ten-minute mile. Six months from now, running at that speed would lower your rate to 145. You know you have to run faster to get the same conditioning effect. Use your target heart rate and get the most from your program.

## SHOULD I EXERCISE WHEN I'M SICK?

Exercising when you're ill is a bad idea. Viral infections are sometimes associated with myocarditis, an inflammation of the heart. Doctors agree exercise is bad for you when you have myocarditis. This condition can lead to heart damage and, in some cases, can cause death. If you have the flu or an illness with a fever, don't exercise until at least several days after the symptoms are gone. When you start again, exercise at a lower intensity. When you are ill, it's much better to rest than to train. Sports and exercise are part of the life process. One purpose of training is to improve your health, not make it worse.

## HOW CAN I ACHIEVE PEAK PERFORMANCE ON A PARTICULAR DAY?

You achieve peak performance by being ready physically and mentally. Physically you want to make sure your muscles have plenty of fuel (glycogen). Your workout schedule during the time preceding the big day is important. You should not have any fatiguing workouts for at least several days prior to the performance. You should increase the carbohydrate content of your diet to maximize muscle glycogen.

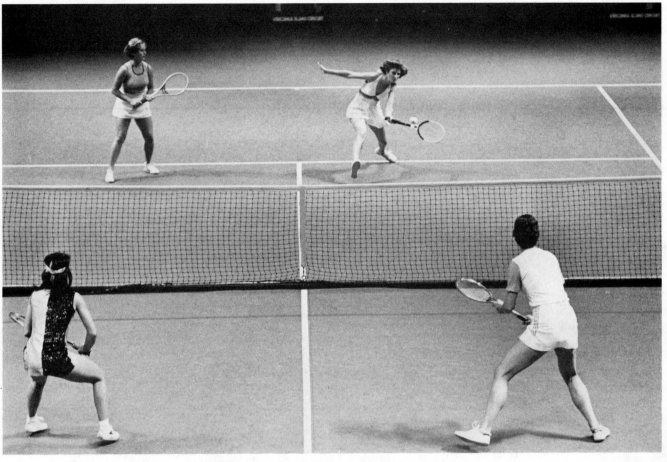

The target heart rate should not be used for stop-and-start games like tennis.

You should sharpen your skills for several weeks. Practice at the speed you will perform. Work on the skills that you're weak in. Break down the components of the performance and think about what you are going to do. Think! A sensible, well-thought-out plan is worth a lot. Your plan should be executed automatically.

Have confidence. If you have prepared yourself to the best of your ability, then you have nothing to be ashamed of. When the time comes put out 100 percent; no—150 percent! As Bear Bryant has said, "My 90 percent ballplayer playing 100 percent will beat your 100 percent ballplayer playing 90 percent every time." Pull out the stops and you'll be awesome. Keep saying "I can." You can and you will!

## WHAT ABOUT SEX AND EXERCISE?

The old adage that sexual intercourse should be avoided before sports performance is false. If you are fit, the energy cost of sex should not affect your play. In fact, sex and exercise are complementary. Exercise gives you fitness for bedroom gymnastics and makes you more appealing to the opposite sex. Sex relaxes you for better exercise performance. Several Olympic athletes have admitted having sex before medal-winning performances. As for the caloric cost of sex, that depends on whether you are a sprinter or an endurance athlete.

## WHAT CAN I DO ABOUT SIDE PAINS DURING RUNNING?

Even the best runners sometimes get side pains (also called a stitch). The exact cause is not known. Sports scientists have speculated that the pains may be caused by gas originating from your intestines. Your diaphragm, a large breathing muscle, may also not be getting enough oxygen and may be going into spasm. The pain is short-lived and usually disappears after you have rested for a while.

There are many things you can try when these pains occur. First, just try "biting the bullet." Sometimes the pain will go away by itself. Resting for a few minutes helps some people; often the pain will be gone when you start up again. Belly breathing, taking deep breaths while running, has been suggested as a possible remedy. Some experts suggest forcefully exhaling against pursed lips while bending at the waist. Having an adequate bowel movement before exercising may be of help if your pains are gas related. Your physician may be able to prescribe an antispasmodic if the pains become too severe.

Pains in the center of your chest or in the neck, shoulders, and arms may be symptomatic of angina pectoris. Angina is caused by a relative lack of blood flow through the coronary arteries, which supply your heart with blood. Don't take any chances; severe chest pains may be a sign of trouble. A man who came through my laboratory had experienced severe chest pains during exercise for several years. He attributed this to a muscle pull in his chest, which he got while chopping wood. It turned out that he had severe heart disease. If you have recurring chest pains during exercise, see your physician.

## SHOULD I TRAIN WHEN IT'S SMOGGY?

Smog, unfortunately, is part of urban life. It is undoubtedly a contributor to various types of cancer and lung diseases. Unless you plan to move to a smogless environment, you had better learn to live with it. Regular endurance exercise is necessary for maintenance of a healthy respiratory system that is capable of high levels of function and can adequately clear pollution products from your system. It's better to be fit than unfit—whether there is smog or not. However, it's probably better not to exercise during a heavy smog alert. High levels of the primary pollutants, carbon monoxide, sulfur dioxide, ozone, and nitrogen dioxide, will decrease your performance and may produce severe respiratory distress. If you are a smoker, the problem is compounded. Exercising during an alert compounds the dangers of smog because by breathing harder, more pollutants enter your system. I played two hours of tennis against a machine several summers ago during a smog alert. I had a lot of trouble breathing comfortably for about five hours after that.

Smog levels are usually lower early in the morning or late at night. If it's smoggy, try to avoid training during the rush hours.

## BODY BEAUTIFUL

The majority of questions people ask me concern body composition and weight control. I never really understood how serious people were about their weight until I got several complaints about the messages my computer was generating about body fat. I had programmed the computer to print out "lose some weight, fatty" if the person was overweight; or "lean and mean" if the person had a desirable fat percentage. Fat is serious business. I believe it's impossible to keep your fat down consistently unless you exercise. I have never seen a crash dieter keep the weight off for very long unless exercise was an important part of the picture. If you understand a few basic principles, you will find body fat management much easier.

## WILL EXERCISE INCREASE MY APPETITE?

On the contrary, moderate levels of exercise actually depress the appetite. I advise people who overindulge at dinner to do their endurance exercise immediately before. This type of exercise channels the blood away from your digestive organs and seems to depress hunger sensations. Athletes, who may burn up to 5,000 calories a day, do need more food, so their appetite increases. My assistant laboratory director is a bicycle road racer. He is a human garbage disposal and the envy of overeaters everywhere. He eats everything in sight but has little body fat. He can eat all he wants because of the calories he burns up on his bicycle.

Dropping your exercise program during a diet is like "throwing the baby out with the bathwater." Crash diets without exercise will help you to lose weight. But, what kind of weight? We have found that much of the weight loss is muscle mass. Body fat management has to involve exercise. When you exercise, you will gain muscle weight and lose fat weight. So, the effect on your actual body weight may not be that noticeable. Your weight loss may be less, but that roll won't protrude over your belt or you'll be able to fit into that smaller dress size. Don't judge your weight control program by scale weight alone. Look at yourself in the mirror. With consistent exercise and diet, you can be thinner.

## HOW DO I LOSE FAT CELLS?

You don't! There are two factors that determine your total amount of body fat: the number and the size of your fat cells. Your total number of fat cells is fixed once you're an adult. After you've stopped growing, you only affect the size of the cells, not the number. You develop the number of fat cells throughout your growing period, but particularly during your first few years of life. It's important to stress good nutrition and exercise habits early. If you can prevent the proliferation of fat cells, body fat will be less of a problem during adulthood. The fat baby may be the obese adult.

Fat cells are involved in the process of maintaining body balance. Remember, the function of a fat cell is to store fat. During crash diets your fat cells are rapidly depleted of fat. These cells react, and other parts of your body are affected. In a study by Dr. D.A. Thompson that appeared in the *Journal of Applied Physiology*, food actually tasted better to people on a starvation diet (crash diets are a type of starvation). Your body reacts to radical attempts to alter its balance. If you go on a sensible, long-term program, you will lose weight and keep it off. Become process oriented. Learn to make exercise and dietary modification a regular part of your life, and you'll stay out of "Fat City."

## ARE RUBBER SUITS EFFECTIVE FOR WEIGHT CONTROL?

Rubber suits and belly bands are a waste of time. There are three components of your body composition that can account for changes in body weight:

1. Body Fat
2. Muscle Mass
3. Body Fluids

Rubber suits cause you to increase your sweat rate. You will lose weight, but it's water weight. Your body closely regulates its fluid balance. As soon as you drink some water, that weight will go right back on. Work on your fat, not your fluid balance.

Altering your body fluids trying to lose weight is foolish and potentially dangerous. Dehydration may lead to heat stroke or heat exhaustion. You may also develop an electrolyte imbalance that could affect your heart's ability to beat or bring about severe muscle cramps. Weight control involves altering your body composition. Changes in body fat are more significant than changes in your body weight.

## HOW CAN I DEVELOP A NICE BODY?

You can develop a nice body by decreasing your body fat and firming up your muscle mass. Much of your body fat lies just underneath the skin on top of your muscles. All the firming in the world will do little to affect that fat layer.

Spot reducing, doing exercises to lose fat in a specific area, is largely a myth. Although a recent study demonstrated that some spot reducing occurs, it is relatively insignificant. The best way to lose body fat is by altering your energy balance: Burn up more calories than you're taking in.

Developing a nice body takes a lot of work, but you can do it. Endurance exercise will help you to develop good muscle tone and at the same time maintain a negative energy balance. The "Total Jock" firming exercises will help you to firm up those muscles. An attractive body results from reducing body fat and firming up your muscles.

## FROM HAND TO MOUTH

America is overrun with food faddists. There are times when I think two-thirds of the population must live near my laboratory. Health food salespeople bombard local athletic teams with the latest elixir to bring instant victory. People are persuaded to use megadoses of vitamins with no other evidence than "if a little is good, a lot must be better." When you ask for scientific evidence, you get the answer, "The AMA is covering up research findings to keep people from getting healthy." If you know some good principles of nutrition, you can improve your performance and at the same time keep down the cost of your urine by consuming fewer food supplements. The burden of proof lies with the food faddists.

## Do I Need More Protein When I Train?

Unless you are involved in super-heavy levels of weight lifting, you don't need any more protein than anyone else. Your protein requirement is about one gram per kilogram body weight per day. In competitive weight lifters the protein requirement has been shown to be about 50 percent higher than this.

Contrary to popular opinion, protein plays a relatively small part in meeting the energy demands of your body during exercise. You can't increase your muscle mass by increasing the protein content of your diet. After your body has all the protein (amino acids) it needs, the rest is converted to fat. Those protein supplements are a pretty expensive way of putting fat on your body.

You do, however, have a minimum protein requirement. If it is not met, your performance will suffer. In addition to making up the structural material of muscle, proteins are important for providing structural materials for metabolic enzymes. These enzymes are important for breaking down fuels for energy during exercise. Particularly if you're a vegetarian, you have to make sure you're eating enough protein. Basic protein groups for vegetarians are eggs, milk products, grains, legumes, nuts, and seeds. The following are some specific examples of protein sources for vegetarians:

1. Eggs
2. Milk
3. Cheeses
4. Soybeans
5. Other beans
6. Seeds (sunflower, pumpkin, sesame)
7. Nuts (cashews, Brazil, peanuts)
8. Wheat germ
9. Barley
10. Bran
11. Spinach
12. Cauliflower
13. Brussels sprouts
14. Brewers yeast

## What Are Anabolic Steroids?

Anabolic steroids are chemicals synthesized in a laboratory to mimic the effects of male hormones. These hormones have two principle actions:

1. To develop male secondary sexual characteristics.
2. To develop muscle mass.

Anabolic steroids have been developed to have the maximum effect on muscle. They are used by many athletes to increase body weight and strength. In some sports such as discus, shotput, and weight lifting, the vast majority of athletes use steroids. There have been allegations that some female athletes from several countries in Europe have also used these drugs.

Several questions are raised:

1. Are these drugs good for you?
2. Do they improve performance?
3. Is it a good idea to fool around with these substances?

Anabolic steroids have some potentially serious side effects. They may be toxic to the liver, and in some people they may be related to the development of prostate or liver cancer. In adolescents they may prematurely stop the growth of long bones. They are also associated with acne and abnormal hair growth. In some people they may drastically affect sperm production. In women they may produce masculinization.

The effectiveness of these steroids in improving athletic performance is controversial. They appear to be beneficial to athletes who train very hard and take protein supplements. I've studied the effects of these drugs on untrained males. These men didn't train very hard, and the drugs had no effect on their muscle mass, strength, or endurance.

I don't think it's a good idea to experiment with these drugs. First, they probably won't do you that much good. And second, you are exposing yourself to a potential health risk.

## Do I Need More Vitamins When I Train?

The only commonly documented dietary deficiency in this country is iron. A large number of women, because of monthly blood loss, are anemic. This anemia can very likely reduce physical performance. The minimum daily requirement of iron for women is 18 milligrams per day. This is somewhat less than the average woman consumes, so a supplement may be needed.

Vitamin C supplementation is very popular with large segments of the population. Prevention and treatment of the common cold are the primary reasons most people take the vitamin. However, little definitive evidence exists to support these claims. Many leading physicians recommend Vitamin C supplements to their patients. In moderate doses, the vitamin is not dangerous. Even if it acts only as a placebo, little harm is done.

Vitamin E is another extremely popular vitamin. Vitamin E is used to prevent heart disease, increase endurance and sexual potency, and as a deodorant. Again, none of these claims have been substantiated. Scientists have found it almost impossible to produce a diet deficient in Vitamin E.

Save your money. You can spend a fortune on vitamins. Instead, spend this money on lift tickets, tennis lessons, running shoes, or a new pair of sweats.

## Are Carbohydrates Important in My Diet?

Carbohydrates are the most important fuel for muscular work. When your carbohydrates run out, your level of performance drops dramatically. Many of the symptoms commonly associated with overtraining—poor performances, chronic tiredness, a dead feeling in your muscles—can sometimes be directly related to lack of carbohydrate stores in your muscles and liver.

High-protein, low-carbohydrate diets have become very popular recently for losing weight. These diets are counterproductive. Your exercise capacity will decrease tremendously without carbohydrates. Exercise is an important means of controlling body weight. Remember, a calorie is a calorie regardless of whether the source is carbohydrate or protein. A successful weight control program has to be process oriented. Short-term goal diets will not keep the weight off. Any weight control program that doesn't involve exercise will ultimately fail.

The "Total Jock" should be on a high-performance diet. This diet should contain at least 50 percent carbohydrate. Don't confuse percentage with total calories. A potato is high in carbohydrates. When you load it up with sour cream and butter, the relative contribution of carbohydrates to total calories becomes low. If you are active, you need carbohydrates. They're the fuel that keeps you going. The following are examples of carbohydrates:

1. Grains
2. Cereals
3. Honey
4. Fruits
5. Breads
6. Noodles
7. Sugar
8. Milk
9. Flour
10. Potatoes
11. Corn

## What's a Good Pre-exercise Meal?

Many good possibilities exist for the pre-exercise meal. Just remember some simple guidelines:

1. Keep the meal low in fat and high in carbohydrates.
2. Eat the meal at least 1½ hours before exercising.
3. Eat something you enjoy.

Meals higher in carbohydrates are relatively easy to digest. You don't want a fatty meal sitting in your digestive system when you are trying to train. Avoid foods with extremely high sugar content immediately before exercise. This will stimulate the secretion of the hormone insulin. Insulin will cause a lowering of blood sugar; that quick energy you hoped to get will backfire on you. But if you eat several hours before training, the insulin effect will subside.

The meals you generally eat are more significant than any pre-exercise meal. Remember, carbohydrate is the high-performance food. Diet possibilities are endless. There are successful athletes in all parts of the globe. They have a great variety of diets. Even though the substance of the diets is different, the principles are the same. Stay away from the big steak as a pre-game meal. That type of meal takes a long time to digest and may harm your performance. A good example of a pre-game meal would be:

1. Toast
2. Juice
3. Nonfat milk

## Is Water Important for Exercise?

Water is one of the most important substances in your body. If you don't have enough of it, your exercise capacity will suffer. Water is used by your body to transport various substances in your blood, to help your cells conduct chemical reactions, and to maintain your body temperature. Even small changes in your body water supply will hurt your capacity to exercise.

Most people don't drink enough water. I've seen people lose five pounds during a jogging session. You should learn to take water breaks. Ideally you should replace your lost water weight at regular intervals. This will have a significant effect on your training. Force yourself to drink a little more water than you need. A good rule of thumb for runners is to attempt to drink about half a pint of water for every 15 minutes of exercise. This should be increased if the air temperature is high. You can learn to recognize when your body temperature is getting too high. If you begin to feel a throbbing pressure in your temples and a cold sensation over your upper body, this may mean that your body temperature is getting too high. The best thing to do is stop exercising and cool down your body gradually.

Water is the best fluid replacement. Many of the commercially available fluid replacements are too high in sugar and electrolytes. Electrolytes are salts such as sodium and potassium. The high sugar content in some of these products slows down the time it takes for water to get into your system. The high electrolyte concentration will actually lead to a type of dehydration. To replace fluids, drink water—the cheapest and the most effective way.

## Should I Take Salt Pills?

I've seen X-rays of intact salt pills sitting in the stomach several hours after being consumed. Salt replacement during exercise is unnecessary and can actually be counterproductive. Too much salt can actually cause parts of your body to dehydrate. You have three basic fluid compartments:

1. Your blood
2. Fluid outside the cells
3. Fluid inside the cells

During exercise there's a shift of fluid toward the inside of cells. This helps to make chemical reactions go faster. When you take in salt during exercise (salt pills or commercial fluid replacements) you cause an increased concentration of the blood (osmolality). Fluid is literally sucked out of the cells. This causes dehydration in an area that critically needs fluid.

Your kidneys are finely tuned to maintain the proper electrolyte balance (salt, potassium). You should be more concerned with taking in enough fluid. Forget about salt; your kidneys will take care of that. As long as the salt content in your diet is adequate, you need no additional supplements.

## WOMEN AND EXERCISE

Before the 1970's there was no widespread participation of women in exercise programs. Many women were embarrassed to jog. In schools, women's athletic programs were few and far between. There was systematic discrimination in women's use of athletic facilities. New laws are providing women with the same athletic opportunities as men. Millions of women now regularly jog, play tennis, swim, and ride bicycles. Physiologists have found the exercise capacity of women is far beyond what was generally believed.

## Does Menstruation Affect Exercise Performance?

The majority of research available indicates that menstruation does not affect exercise performance. In fact, active women have fewer headaches and fewer symptoms of premenstrual tension. However, under certain circumstances heavy training can affect the menstrual cycle. In the United States, athletes tend to have their first period later than non-athletes. This is particularly true for endurance sports such as distance running. Dr. Ken Forman, Olympic women's distance running coach, has found that many runners have irregular menstrual periods. This seems to be related to the runners' total body fat. When fat is less than 16 percent of total weight, menstrual periods sometimes become irregular. This may account for the delay in menarche experienced in female athletes—menstruation is delayed because they don't develop the fat typical for adolescent girls.

## Can You Exercise During Pregnancy?

Pregnant women can perform endurance exercise. A woman in Dallas ran five miles per day until three weeks before giving birth, with no apparent ill effects to the baby or herself. The fetus is well protected from jarring and injuries. Pregnant women should probably not exercise at extremely high intensities because of the possibility of decreasing the oxygen supply to the unborn child. Regular exercise is helpful in preventing back pains that typically accompany pregnancy. There is not a tremendous amount of information available yet on how much exercise is good, so it's best simply to follow the advice of your obstetrician.

## What Accounts for Performance Differences Between Men and Women?

Men generally have a higher exercise capacity than women because of their body size. The greater male muscle mass results in higher levels of strength. In addition, men generally have a greater capacity to transport oxygen because of their larger heart size and more hemoglobin (which carries oxygen). Physiologically, the differences are caused by the male hormone testosterone, which is present in about ten times greater amount in adult males than in adult females. Before puberty, when testosterone levels are similar in boys and girls, there is little difference in exercise capacity. During adolescence, higher levels of male hormones result in increasing muscle mass, strength, and work capacity in males.

There is considerable overlap in exercise performance. Athletic records set by men in the early 1960's are now being matched by women in several sports. Women have been very successful in extremely long road races greater than 50 miles, beating male competitors. Women may have a greater capacity to use fats over long periods of time. In any event, a trained woman can participate with trained men in any sport at a recreational level.

Women tend to excel in sports requiring balance because of a lower center of gravity. Women are more efficient in swimming because their higher fat percentage causes less resistance in the water. If women had the same cardiovascular capacity as men, they would produce superior performances. In addition, women are generally more flexible than men, which makes them less susceptible to certain types of injury.

## Do Women Get Large Muscles from Exercise?

Any muscle, if exercised heavily over a long period of time, will get larger. Women develop muscle at a much slower rate than men. Even years of exhaustive training, such as swimming, will not produce the degree of muscle hypertrophy (enlargement) seen in men. The male hormone testosterone is the most important factor associated with muscle enlargement. Women just don't have high enough levels of testosterone to get big muscles.

Weight training, an activity associated with bulging biceps and Mr. America, is becoming a popular sport with women across the country. Sports scientists have shown that weight training results in loss of body fat with only modest increases in muscle tissue. This type of exercise in women results in increases in strength with little effect on size. You don't have to worry about looking like Hercules Unchained. Weight training will help you develop a nice body while increasing your strength for sports.

# SCIENCE AND EXERCISE

## How will Exercise Science Affect the Average Person in the Years to Come?

Science will play an increasing role in helping you with your sporty lifestyle. New and better equipment will be developed to make exercise safer and more enjoyable. Scientific advances in sports medicine are moving at a fantastic rate. Many of these advances have been due to the computer. New discoveries will help the average person as well as the athlete.

Ten years ago metabolic measurement in exercising humans was an extremely tedious undertaking. Gases were collected in large cumbersome canvas bags and then analyzed chemically by procedures that were long and difficult. A single treadmill test took several hours. With computers and high-speed gas analyzers, metabolic calculations now can be made instantly. Precise metabolic measurements and computerized exercise prescription are available for everyone. The cost is modest. We now have the capacity to give a person a running speed that will result in the fastest possible progress.

Computers will also make the science of biomechanics available to the average person. Biomechanics is the study of movement; movements are studied for efficiency. In the future high-speed film will be analyzed by computer. Your technique will be broken down into its components. You will know precisely what to do for maximum improvement. Athletes now use biomechanics to win gold medals. You will be able to use it to improve your tennis game or clean up your running style.

New methods of gaining strength have already arrived. The most promising of these are isokinetic devices that train your muscles to exert more force at fast speeds of movement. These new devices will develop strength that you can use in sports.

In the field of psychology, we will also have many contributions. Psychologists will teach you new methods of selecting the sports you're most suited for. Meditation methods may help you develop the concentration to win.

It's difficult for women to develop large muscles from exercise.

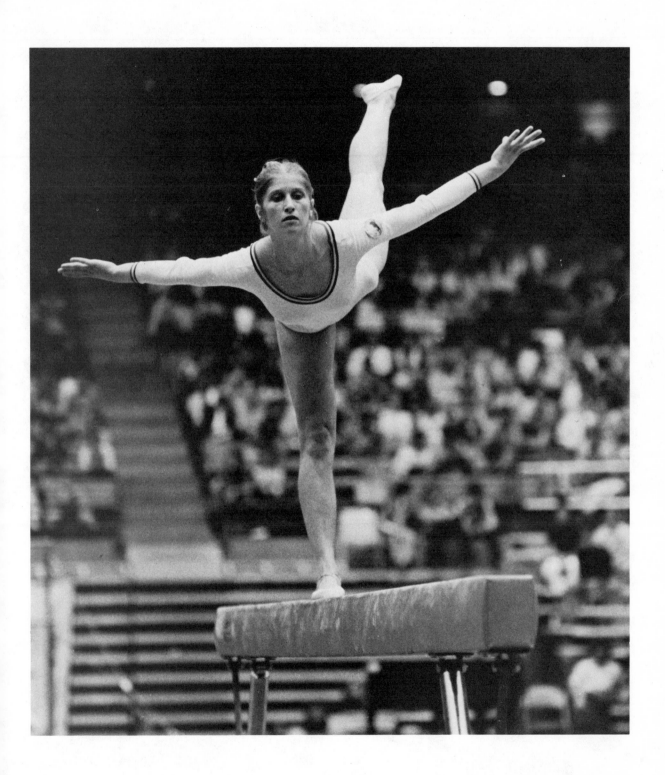

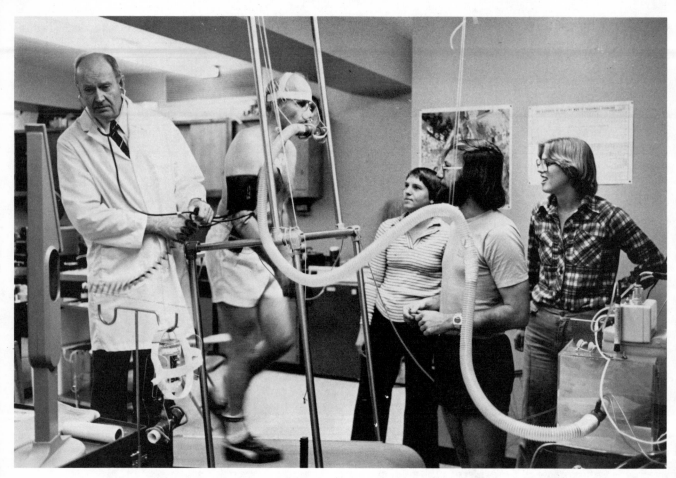
The treadmill test

Biochemists will determine if you're more suited for endurance or speed exercise. You can use this information to go into the activities where you're likely to find success.

Science will help you in many ways, but it's up to you to lead the active life. I am reminded of an old Viking drinking toast, "Skaal ska du ha, Godt skal du faa, men so skal due selv ver umde." Translated, this roughly means, "Cheers to you all, the best of luck, but you must do something for yourself."

## INSTANT REPLAY

1. To improve your fitness you must continue to increase the training load. This is the overload principle.
2. You can avoid injury by progressing slowly and putting yourself in top physical condition. Make sure you warm up adequately before exercise and warm down when you finish training.
3. Never exercise when you are ill.
4. Your target heart rate for endurance exercise will be between 70 and 85 percent of your maximum heart rate. You can estimate your maximum heart rate by subtracting your age from the number 220.
5. To lose fat you must use more calories than you take in.
6. Carbohydrates are an important fuel for exercise. Make sure your diet contains at least 50 percent carbohydrates.
7. Women will not get large muscles from exercise. Women do not develop muscle as rapidly as men because they do not have high levels of male hormones.

# CHAP4TER

# HIGHER, FASTER, FURTHER:
## Assessing Your Fitness

**S**hin splints, sore legs, aching ankles, cramps . . . "I've got to run seven minutes a mile. My aching back. How long is it going to take me to get in shape? Exercise doesn't make you live longer, it just seems longer."

Why do exercise and pain always seem to go together? The reason is simple: Most people do too much too soon. You can become well conditioned and fit if you increase your training intensity progressively. You don't need to be so tired after your workout that you have a sick feeling in the pit of your stomach and your legs cry out for mercy. You can minimize the discomfort of exercise if you know your capacity and systematically build your body's fitness in small steps.

In this chapter I'm going to help you discover where you are in your quest for the sporting life. I have provided some simple tests that will help you determine your maximum metabolic capacity (max mets). I will also help you assess your ability to participate in a variety of sports that are the backbone of the activity-oriented existence. With these simple tests, you will have a pretty good idea of where you stand. In later chapters I will show you how to systematically improve your sports skills, endurance, strength, flexibility, and speed.

## MAX METS

Endurance is a common denominator for all sports. Even in sports with low energy requirements, such as golf and bowling, your metabolic capacity has an effect on your success. If you have a poor work capacity, you will tire rapidly and your performance will suffer. I have provided five methods of measuring your max mets or endurance capacity:

1. One-mile walk
2. Three-mile walk
3. 1½-mile run
4. Three-mile bicycle ride
5. 400-yard swim

Your results may differ radically on each test. This is due to the metabolic specificity of each activity. Physiologically your body reacts somewhat differently to running, swimming, and bicycling. You can be fit for one type of exercise and not another; this is metabolic specificity.

Use the running test to gauge your fitness capacity for sports. This type of exercise stress best measures your readiness for most sports. The swimming and cycling tests have been provided to help you measure your capacity for training in the swimming pool or on a bicycle.

If you are over 35 years of age, I strongly urge you to get a physical examination, including a stress electrocardiogram. The number of people running around with undiagnosed heart disease is frightening. Training may be difficult in the hereafter. If you haven't been exercising regularly, start with the walking tests. If you've been jogging 4½ miles per week or more for at least six weeks, start with the running test.

## WALKING TEST

Find a flat area with a known length. A 440-yard running track is probably the best. You can also use your car's odometer to help you measure a course around your neighborhood.

### One-Mile Walk

Walk one mile as fast as you can. Try to keep your pace constant during the entire test. Don't start off slow and finish fast. The met values correspond to the following mile-walk times. The met value of your mile time is the number of times you have to increase your metabolism above rest.

### ONE-MILE WALK

| Your Time | Mets (Approximate Metabolic Cost) |
|-----------|-----------------------------------|
| 30 minutes | 2.5 |
| 25 minutes | 2.9 |
| 20 minutes | 3.3 |
| 19 minutes | 3.4 |
| 18 minutes | 3.6 |
| 17 minutes | 3.7 |
| 16 minutes | 3.9 |
| 15 minutes | 4.1 |

If you can complete the mile in less than 15 minutes, then you can take the three-mile walk test. If you walk the mile in less than 15 minutes, you have a max mets of at least 4. This means that you can increase your metabolism at least four times above rest.

If you fail to finish this test in less than 15 minutes, repeat the test every day until you can. Failure to walk a mile in less than 15 minutes indicates a very low level of fitness. I strongly urge you to see your doctor and to join a structured exercise class. Independent exercise may be dangerous for you.

## Three-Mile Walk

This time walk three miles as fast as you can. The met cost for a 15 minute mile is still 4.1. This test measures the ability to increase your metabolism to levels required in moderate level sports and keep it there. The 3-mile walk cutoff time is 45 minutes.

If you can't make the 45-minute cutoff but made 15 minutes in the one-mile walk, then you need to go on a walking program before you can take the running test. You can use the 3-mile walking test as a conditioner. Repeat this test three to five times a week until you reach the target time. Be sure to do the flexibility exercises shown in Chapter 7 before each walk. After you have successfully completed the three-mile walk in less than 45 minutes, you are ready to prepare for the 1½ mile run.

## 1½-MILE RUN TEST

The 1½-mile run test will be used to calculate your max mets. If you haven't been running at least 4½ miles a week for six weeks or more, complete the 1½-mile preparation program before taking the test. This program is designed to introduce your body gradually to the rigors of running. The program takes roughly five weeks and requires four to five days per week. Do not proceed to the next week until you can complete the present weeks' workouts. Don't worry about an extra week or so.

Before taking this test, warm up thoroughly. Do your stretching exercises, and walk and jog for several minutes before beginning.

| Week | Workout | Days per Week |
|:---:|:---|:---:|
| 1 | 1½ miles: alternate walking 50 yards, jogging 50 yards. Stretch before and after workout (see Chapter 7) | 4 |
| 2 | 2 miles: alternate jogging 100 yards, walking 100 yards. Stretch before and after | 5 |
| 3 | 2 miles: alternate jogging 300 yards, walking 100 yards. Stretch before and after | 5 |
| 4 | 2 miles: alternate jogging 400–600 yards, walking 100 yards. Stretch before and after | 4–5 |
| 5 | 2 miles: jogging as far as you can, walking 100 yards, jog-walk remainder of 2 miles. Stretch before and after | 4–5 |

Remember, your heart needs to be warmed up as well as your muscles. It's best to take this test on a 440-yard track.

Run the 1½-mile run as fast as you can, but try to keep your running speed the same throughout the test. Determine your max mets from the 1½-mile run table. You can use your max mets to assess your fitness for sports by referring to the Met Table later in this chapter. In addition, your max mets are used to determine your starting point in the running and walking program shown in Chapter 5.

The 1½-mile run test is a good way to assess your metabolic capacity. By taking this test from time to time, you can measure your progress. Ideally, you should have your capacity assessed on a treadmill, but you will find the 1½-mile run a pretty good substitute.

## 1½-MILE RUN TEST

| Time Min:Sec | Your Max Mets |
|:---:|:---:|
| 8:05 | 18.0 |
| 8:20 | 17.5 |
| 8:35 | 17.0 |

## 1½-MILE RUN TEST

| Time<br>Min:Sec | Your Max Mets |
|:---:|:---:|
| 8:55 | 16.5 |
| 9:10 | 16.0 |
| 9:31 | 15.5 |
| 9:50 | 15.0 |
| 10:16 | 14.5 |
| 10:35 | 14.0 |
| 11:01 | 13.5 |
| 11:31 | 13.0 |
| 12:01 | 12.5 |
| 12:35 | 12.0 |
| 13:10 | 11.5 |
| 13:50 | 11.0 |
| 14:31 | 10.5 |
| 15:20 | 10.0 |
| 16:10 | 9.5 |
| 17:16 | 9.0 |
| 18:25 | 8.5 |
| 19:40 | 8.0 |
| 21:16 | 7.5 |

## THREE-MILE BICYCLE TEST

Use the bicycle test to determine your max mets for the bicycle exercise program shown in the next chapter. Your max mets on a bicycle will vary with the type of bicycle, your cycling skill, and your body weight. However, the major determinant of energy cost on a bicycle is speed. The faster you go, the higher the energy cost. Your cycling program should be done on the same bicycle on which you took this test. Because of the specificity of exercise, use the running test (1½-mile run) to determine your readiness for sports.

Prepare for the three-mile bike test in a similar manner to the 1½-mile run. If you haven't been riding a bicycle regularly for at least six weeks, complete the preliminary bicycle exercise program before taking the test.

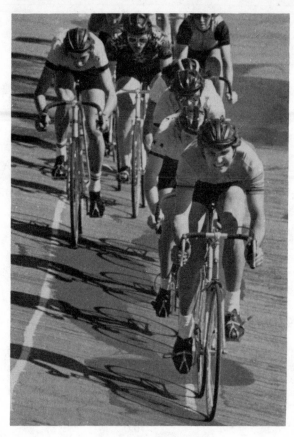

Bicycling:
your speed is the most important
factor in determining the energy cost.

## Preparing for the Three-Mile Bicycle Test

Try to ride in an area with minimal traffic congestion. A good endurance program requires that you sustain a relatively high heart rate for at least 20 minutes. It takes time to build up to this. Complete the preparatory program before taking the test.

| Week | Workout | Days per Week |
|------|---------|---------------|
| 1 | Ride 5 minutes | 4 |
| 2 | Ride 10 minutes (Increase pace a little) | 5 |
| 3 | Ride 15 minutes | 4–5 |
| 4 | Ride 20 minutes | 4–5 |

The preparation for cycling is not as important as for running. In running, you have to contend with the forces of gravity. Because cycling is basically a non-weight-bearing activity, the risk of injury is less.

After you have prepared your body for the rigors of an all-out bicycle ride, you have to find a flat area that's suitable for the test. The best place is a bicycle track. There are few tracks around, so the next best place is a quiet residential section of town with little traffic. In the city, a large park may have a good place to ride continuously for three miles. As a last resort, a running track may be suitable. Avoid the people who maintain the running track, or the three-mile test may be your last ride.

During the test, ride as fast as you can. Try to keep the pace consistent throughout the ride. Use your time to determine your max mets for bicycling. You can use your bicycle max mets to help you choose a starting point for the bicycle training program shown in the next chapter.

### THREE-MILE BICYCLE TEST

| Time Min:Sec | Your Max Mets |
|---|---|
| 5:53 | 20.0 |
| 6:00 | 19.5 |
| 6:08 | 19.0 |
| 6:17 | 18.5 |
| 6:26 | 18.0 |
| 6:35 | 17.5 |
| 6:45 | 17.0 |
| 6:55 | 16.5 |
| 7:05 | 16.0 |
| 7:17 | 15.5 |
| 7:29 | 15.0 |
| 7:41 | 14.5 |
| 7:54 | 14.0 |
| 8:08 | 13.5 |
| 8:23 | 13.0 |
| 8:39 | 12.5 |
| 8:56 | 12.0 |
| 9:14 | 11.5 |
| 9:33 | 11.0 |
| 9:54 | 10.5 |
| 10:16 | 10.0 |
| 10:40 | 9.5 |
| 11:05 | 9.0 |
| 11:33 | 8.5 |
| 12:04 | 8.0 |
| 12:37 | 7.5 |
| 13:13 | 7.0 |

## THREE-MILE BICYCLE TEST

| Time Min:Sec | Your Max Mets |
|---|---|
| 13:53 | 6.5 |
| 14:37 | 6.0 |
| 15:26 | 5.5 |
| 16:21 | 5.0 |

# 400-YARD SWIM TEST

The mets determined from the swim test only apply to swimming. Mets are used very loosely when applied to swimming exercise. In swimming, speed is affected by such factors as the efficiency of your strokes and your drag in the water. A speed that would require little energy from a world-class swimmer would require a great deal more from an untrained person. Although the term *mets* has a definite basis in metabolic physiology, I am using the term very loosely when talking about swimming. However, because your swimming program is based on your own performance, the progression of your workouts is correct.

As with bicycling, preparation for the swim test is not as critical as in running. You weigh only a few pounds in water and are thus not as susceptible to injury. Beginning swimmers expend a great deal of energy trying to stay level in the water. If you want to use swimming as a conditioner, you have to develop enough skill to swim continuously for 20 to 30 minutes.

If you can't swim, your first task is to learn. The Red Cross, Y's, and most recreation departments are great places to take lessons. Swimming is a good thing to know even if you don't plan to use it for exercise; you never know when you may fall in the drink.

For both your swimming workouts and your test, it's best to use a 25-yard pool. Although a smaller pool is adequate, you spend much of your time pushing off the side. In a smaller pool, you can swim around the perimeter and thus swim continuously for a longer period of time.

If you haven't been swimming regularly, condition yourself before taking the 400-yard test.

| Week | Workout | Days per Week |
|---|---|---|
| 1 | 100–200 yards | 4 |
| 2 | 200–400 yards | 5 |
| 3 | 400–600 yards | 4–5 |
| 4 | 600 yards | 4–5 |

For the test, swim 400 yards as fast as you can. Again, keep the pace as uniform as possible.

### 400-YARD SWIM TEST

| Time<br>Min:Sec | Your Max Mets |
|:---:|:---:|
| 5:41 | 17.0 |
| 5:49 | 16.5 |
| 5:57 | 16.0 |
| 6:05 | 15.5 |
| 6:14 | 15.0 |
| 6:23 | 14.5 |
| 6:32 | 14.0 |
| 6:42 | 13.5 |
| 6:53 | 13.0 |
| 7:04 | 12.5 |
| 7:16 | 12.0 |
| 7:28 | 11.5 |
| 7:41 | 11.0 |
| 7:55 | 10.5 |
| 8:10 | 10.0 |
| 8:26 | 9.5 |
| 8:43 | 9.0 |
| 9:01 | 8.5 |
| 9:20 | 8.0 |
| 9:41 | 7.5 |
| 10:03 | 7.0 |
| 10:27 | 6.5 |
| 10:53 | 6.0 |
| 11:21 | 5.5 |
| 11:52 | 5.0 |
| 12:25 | 4.5 |
| 13:02 | 4.0 |

# SPORTS

In this section you will determine the following:

1. Are you in good enough shape to participate in most sports?
2. Are you skilled in a variety of sports and games?
3. Are there new activities that you would like to learn?

Most people have no idea of the many possibilities that exist for them. Use a little imagination. Do some exploring. There are a lot of activities out there that may be just what you're looking for. New sports become popular all the time. Three perfect examples are racquetball, skateboarding, and aerobic dance.

Ten years ago the closest thing to racquetball was squash, a sport known to relatively few people. All of a sudden, racquetball players started taking over handball and squash courts. The game was a natural for popularity with large numbers of people. You could go out and play and have fun almost immediately. Because you're in a small area, you have a good chance of hitting the ball. There is less of the hit and fetch that is the universal experience of beginning tennis players. I wouldn't miss my weekly racquetball games for anything. I don't even think of it as exercise, even though I'm usually drenched with sweat after the game.

Skateboarding is an unlikely sport for mass popularity. I consider myself a pioneer of skateboarding. In the late 1950's and early 1960's, I would nail old roller skates on the bottom of a board and plummet down the hills of San Francisco. What I did is considered child's play by today's

Skateboarding

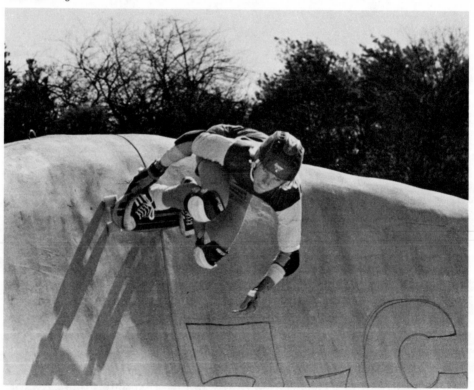

skateboard aficionados. Recently I went to a skateboard park. A skateboard park is a series of cement-covered pits resembling irregularly shaped swimming pools. Modern skateboarders wear helmets, knee and elbow pads, and gloves. They careen down one steep wall and up another. It's an entirely new experience that's a cross between skiing and surfing. It's a perfect sport for the summer and fall when there's no snow in the hills. Because of the risk of serious injury, however, protective equipment is essential. If you're just starting, be careful.

Aerobic dance is another new type of exercise that has been developed to take people's minds off the medicinal aspect of exercise training. It satisfies all of the necessary prerequisites of an endurance exercise: large-muscle, rhythmic exercise that increases the metabolic rate to over 60 percent of maximum for a prolonged period of time. This type of exercise uses dance as a means of developing endurance capacity. Aerobic dancers are encouraged to move to music continuously and at a fast enough rate to get a conditioning effect. Many people prefer this type of exercise because it's fun, yet it still provides them with a regular form of exercise. As you become better conditioned, the dances become more physically demanding. It's conceivable that you could achieve a relatively high level of fitness if you dance vigorously enough.

## The Met Chart

I have prepared a chart to help you assess the extent of your sports involvement. It will help you determine where you are now and where you want to be. I have listed a variety of sports with their met cost and their max met requirement. Remember, the met cost of an activity is its energy cost. Sports requiring a lot of energy have a high met cost. Your max mets are a measure of your maximum energy level or your maximum exercise capacity. The better condition you're in, the higher your max mets. Your max mets should always be higher than the met cost of an activity, the higher the better. Compare your max mets (from the 1½-mile run test) with the minimum max mets requirement of the sport. If you are in good enough condition for the sport, make a check in the column marked "I'm physically prepared." In the column marked "skill level," give yourself a 1 if you are skilled enough to enjoy yourself without additional instruction and are playing up to your expectations; 2 if you need a little more help; 3 if you are a beginner; and 4 if you've never played.

# APPROXIMATE MET COSTS AND FITNESS REQUIREMENTS
## OF SPORTS FOR THE "TOTAL JOCK"

My max mets: _____

| Conditioning Sports | Met Cost | Minimum Max Mets | I'm physically prepared | Skill Level |
|---|---|---|---|---|
| Running (6 minutes per mile) | 16 | 17.5 | | |
| Running (8 minutes per mile) | 13 | 14.5 | | |
| Swimming (2 minutes per 100 yards) (noncompetitive swimmers) | 12 | 13.5 | | |
| Swimming (3 minutes per 100 yards) (noncompetitive swimmers) | 5 | 7.5 | | |
| Bicycling (20 miles per hour) | 12 | 13.5 | | |
| Bicycling (9 miles per hour) | 3.5 | 6 | | |
| Calisthenics (conditioning exercises) | 3–8 | 5–11 | | |
| Stair Climbing | 4–8 | 6.5–11 | | |
| *Mountain Sports** | | | | |
| Downhill Skiing | | | | |
|   Cruising | 5–8 | 9–12 | | |
|   Bumps and Powder | 7–14 | 12–17 | | |
|   Competitive | 12–16 | 14–18 | | |
| Cross-Country Skiing | | | | |
|   Recreational | 6–12 | 11–14.5 | | |
|   Competitive | 10–21 | 17–24 | | |
| Mountain Climbing | 5–10 | 12.5–15 | | |
| Backpacking | 5–11 | 10–14 | | |
| Snow Shoeing | 7–14 | 13–16.5 | | |
| Sledding | 4–8 | 7–10 | | |
| Hunting | | | | |
|   Small Game | 3–7 | 7–10 | | |
|   Big Game | 3–14 | 7–16 | | |
| White Water Kayaking | 3–8 | 6.5–11.5 | | |
| Fly Fishing | 5–6 | 6–8.5 | | |
| Ice Skating | 5–8 | 8–11.5 | | |
| Snowmobile | 2–4 | 5–6 | | |
| Motorcross (cross country motorcycle) | 6–10 | 10–14 | | |

*Altitude must be taken into consideration. Although met cost of an activity will be the same at all elevations, the higher the altitude, the more your maximum capacity decreases. Your max mets will decrease 3 percent every 1,000 feet above 6,000 feet.

| Conditioning Sports | Met Cost | Minimum Max Mets | I'm physically prepared | Skill Level |
|---|---|---|---|---|
| Orienteering (cross country in mountains on foot) | 10–20 | 16–22 | | |
| Horseback Riding | 3–8 | 5–11.4 | | |
| *Water Sports* | | | | |
| Scuba and Skin Diving | 5–12 | 8–14 | | |
| Water Volleyball | 3–8 | 5–11 | | |
| Fishing | | | | |
|   From Boat or Bank | 2–4 | 4–5.5 | | |
|   Big Game | 2–7 | 4–10 | | |
| Water Skiing | 5–7 | 8–10 | | |
| Body Surfing | 4–7 | 6.5–10 | | |
| Board Surfing | 4–7 | 6.5–10 | | |
| Sailing | 2–5 | 3.5–7.5 | | |
| Canoeing and Rowing | 3–8 | 5–12 | | |
| *Competitive Sports* | | | | |
| Badminton | 4–9 | 6.5–13 | | |
| Basketball | | | | |
|   Half Court | 3–9 | 5–13 | | |
|   Full Court | 7–12 | 12–14 | | |
| Handball | 8–12 | 13–14 | | |
| Racquetball | 8–12 | 13–14 | | |
| Squash | 8–12 | 13–14 | | |
| Softball | 3–6 | 5–8.5 | | |
| Table Tennis | 3–5 | 5–7 | | |
| Tennis | 4–9 | 7–13 | | |
| Volleyball | 3–6 | 5–8.5 | | |
| Gymnastics | 3–5 | 5–7 | | |
| *Social Sports* | | | | |
| Boogie Dancing | 3–8 | 5–11.5 | | |
| Square Dancing | 3–7 | 5–10 | | |
| Golf | | | | |
|   Power Cart | 2–3 | 4–5 | | |
|   Walking | 4–7 | 7–10 | | |
| Roller Skating | 5–8 | 8–11.5 | | |
| Horseshoes | 2–3 | 4–5 | | |
| Shuffleboard | 2–3 | 4–5 | | |
| Archery | 3–4 | 5–6 | | |
| Bowling | 2–4 | 4–6 | | |

## Fitness Level

The more fit you are, the more sports you can play. Fit people can play harder and longer and with fewer injuries. Ideally, your max mets should be greater than 13 or 14, regardless of your age. If your max mets are less than 10, then you definitely need to improve your fitness level. The fitness program in Chapter 5 will prepare you rapidly for sports. Remember, you have to work on fitness regularly. You can't work hard for a few months and expect to have a high capacity for the rest of your life. It just doesn't happen like that.

Having a high max mets is not the total answer to fitness. You have to develop strength, speed, and flexibility. In addition, as you develop your sports skills, you become more efficient; you expend less energy. You must develop all-around fitness.

## Sports Skills

If you have mostly 4's on your list, then it's time to learn some new skills. The more sports you know, the more fun you'll have. In the last chapter I'll tell you a few gimmicks to help you maintain the enthusiasm of an athlete about to participate in the Olympic Games.

Make a commitment to yourself. There are few sports that you're not capable of enjoying. If you're like me, you'll probably want to try all the sports you've never tried before. Establish priorities. Write down the five sports you want to learn most, and go out and try them.

**SPORTS I'M GOING TO LEARN**

1.
2.
3.
4.
5.

## Skill Level

In Chapter 8, I'll show you ways to increase your skill in any activity. Don't compare your skill level with anyone else. It's a shame when people don't try a sport because they feel they aren't skilled enough. Gauge your skill level by your enjoyment. If more skill will increase your enjoyment, then your game needs work. However, if you're having fun where you are, then don't worry about it. Most people don't care what your skill level is. If they do, that's their problem. Let them worry about maintaining their status as the ultra-skilled; you worry about having fun.

You can perceive yourself as successful at any level of skill. See yourself as successful, and you are successful. Thomas Edison tried 1,200 different types of filaments for his light bulb before he found one that worked. A newspaper reporter asked him how it felt to have failed 1,200 times. Edison told the person he hadn't failed; he had found 1,200 different filaments that didn't work.

Make the best of what you have. Don't worry about your natural ability. You can always improve a little. Small improvements over a long period of time add up to monumental achievements. Improving your skill is a small matter. Think about why you can do something, not why you can't.

## Strength, Speed, Flexibility, and Agility

I'm not going to give you any tests to measure these factors. Even though they are very important, it's almost impossible to provide good, accurate tests to determine readiness for sports. I don't know how many pushups you need to be able to do to swim properly. I don't know how much flexibility in your leg muscles is needed to play tennis well. These factors are extremely specific to the activity. The type of strength required in racquetball is different from the strength required in white water rafting.

I worked for several years developing tests to predict the ability to perform physical tasks of police work. After administering many types of tests to hundreds of applicants, I found the best way was for people to do the tasks themselves. The best way to measure your ability to climb a six-foot fence is to climb one. Pushup and situp tests that we all took in physical education classes just don't predict the strength and agility needed in specific activities.

I think it's very important for you to improve your strength, flexibility, and quickness. You will develop these by working in the various sports and by practicing the various types of exercises outlined in the next few chapters.

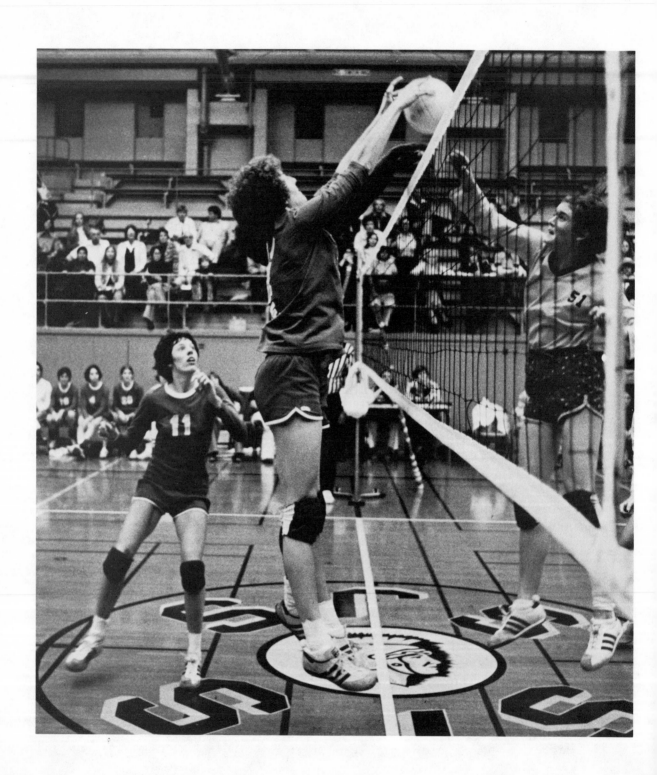

## INSTANT REPLAY

1. Use the 1½-mile run test to determine your max mets for sports.
2. Do not take the 1½-mile run test, the three-mile bicycle test, or the 400-yard swim test until you have completed the preliminary conditioning exercises.
3. The met cost of a sport tells you its energy requirement. Your max mets should be well above the met cost of an activity. You can use the met chart to determine your physical readiness for a sport.
4. Develop a positive attitude about sports. You can be better.

Volleyball: 3–6 mets

# CHAP5TER

# TRAINING FOR ENDURANCE AND SPEED

**M**ovement is what fitness is all about. I'm not just talking about running in a straight line. That's only part of it. I'm talking about using your body in a variety of movements—moving quickly to hit a ball in tennis, moving from one edge to another in skiing, or moving against a current in scuba diving. You have to train your body in a variety of ways to be prepared for the many types of movements. You can increase the efficiency of your movements by playing a variety of sports and by practicing exercises that specifically increase your speed, endurance, strength, and flexibility. In this chapter I'll help you develop better movement by showing you proven methods of developing endurance capacity and the ability to move faster.

## IMPROVING YOUR MAX METS

The best way to improve your max mets is to practice regular endurance exercise. The best and most practical exercises of this kind are running, bicycling, and swimming.

Through the use of a computer, I have developed running, swimming, and cycling programs that will help you improve your max mets. To use these programs, determine your max mets from the tests in the last chapter. Use the 1½-mile run test for the running program, the three-mile bike test for the bicycle program, and the 400-yard swim test for the swimming program. If you haven't progressed beyond the walking tests, continue with your walking program until you are ready for the 1½-mile run test.

To use the charts, find the starting step that corresponds to your max mets. For example, if your max mets is 7 according to the 1½-mile run, you should start at step 9 of the "Total Jock" running program; if your max mets is 8, you start at step 13. To use the bike program, use the bike test to determine your max mets. As with the running program, bikers should start at the step that corresponds to their max mets.

Swimmers use the swimming test and follow the same procedures as runners and bikers. Remain at a step until you can finish the distance in the target time comfortably. As you increase your step position, your fitness will improve. Remember, each step represents a training level that will be between 70 and 85 percent of your max mets. Don't try to progress too fast.

## How Many Days a Week Should I Practice These Exercises?

You should train three to five days a week. Ideally, you should mix up your workouts. For example, you could run three days, ride your bicycle one day, and swim one day. You get different benefits from each program, so a variety is helpful. Some people like to train six to seven days per week. For most people this poses no problem. However, overtraining increases your chances of injury and may result in chronic fatigue.

## When Am I in Good Enough Shape to Level Off?

Most people are unwilling and unable to work at the highest steps of these programs. It is neither necessary nor desirable to keep improving once you have reached an adequate level of fitness. You have reached an adequate level of fitness when you have the endurance capacity to perform the majority of sports activities. Shoot for 13 or 14 mets. Many people want to be more fit than that, and so I have included steps to improve fitness for those who have already achieved high levels of performance.

After you have the fitness you need, continue to exercise at the last step you have attained. Working at that step three to five days a week will keep you there.

## How Long Do I Stay at Each Step?

Stay as long as you have to. These levels are designed to provide an exercise intensity that results in the optimal rate of improvement for you. If the target time is 20 minutes, don't complete the distance in 15 minutes. Your task is to complete the distance in the target time. Improve your fitness slowly and you will progress with a minimum of discomfort. If you have to stay at a step for a month, don't worry about it.

When you can complete the distance in the target time, move to the next step. Your heart rate will also tell you when to progress. When it drops by several beats at a given step, it's time to move on.

Retake the max met tests every three to six months so that you can evaluate your progress and your exercise level.

After you have reached a fitness level you are comfortable with, remain at that step. This way you will maintain your fitness.

## HOW WERE THESE PROGRAMS DERIVED?

These programs were calculated on the basis of the way people improve their fitness capacity. Sports scientists have found you must exercise at a level of at least 60 percent of your maximum capacity to effectively improve your fitness. This program gradually increases the relative intensity of your exercise. In addition, steps are arranged so that you increase the amount of time you can sustain an exercise pace. With this program you consistently improve the intensity of your exercise and the amount of time you can maintain this intensity.

I have selected the minimum effective exercise time for your workouts—20 to 30 minutes. If you wish to train longer, use the informa-

Use the 400-yard swim test to determine your starting level for the swimming program.

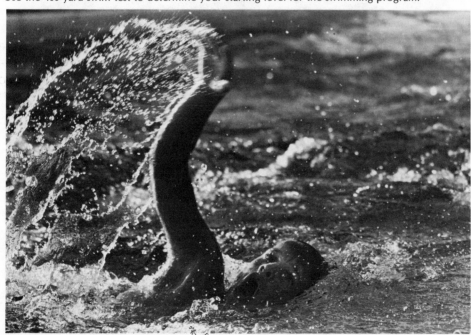

tion in the charts about movement speed to figure out your own program. So, if you want to run for one hour instead of 20 minutes, you can use the appropriate pace to figure out a longer workout.

## WHAT IF I STOP EXERCISING DUE TO ILLNESS OR SOME OTHER REASON?

If you stop exercising for a time, particularly due to illness, go back a few steps and progress gradually. Don't try to go too fast. As a general principle, if you have been ill, you should rest one day for each day you were indisposed before resuming your program. If you start any earlier, you may risk a relapse.

### "TOTAL JOCK" RUNNING PROGRAM

Use 1½-mile run test to determine your max mets. Start at the first step of your max met level. Remain at step until you can complete distance in target time.

| Step | Max Mets | Distance (miles) | Target Time (min:sec) | Speed Minutes/Mile (min:sec) | Pace |
|------|----------|------------------|-----------------------|------------------------------|----------|
| 1 | 5 | 1.0 | 17:42 | 17:42 | Walk-Run |
| 2 | | 1.5 | 25:54 | 17:16 | Walk-Run |
| 3 | | 1.5 | 25:17 | 16:51 | Walk-Run |
| 4 | | 1.5 | 24:41 | 16:27 | Walk-Run |
| 5 | 6 | 2.0 | 33:02 | 16:31 | Walk-Run |
| 6 | | 1.5 | 24:06 | 16:04 | Walk-Run |
| 7 | | 1.5 | 23:28 | 15:38 | Walk-Run |
| 8 | | 1.5 | 22:51 | 15:14 | Walk-Run |
| 9 | 7 | 2.0 | 30:56 | 15:28 | Walk-Run |
| 10 | | 1.5 | 22:30 | 15:00 | Walk-Run |
| 11 | | 1.5 | 21:51 | 14:34 | Walk-Run |
| 12 | | 1.5 | 21:14 | 14:09 | Walk-Run |
| 13 | 8 | 2.0 | 29:01 | 14:30 | Walk-Run |
| 14 | | 1.5 | 21:04 | 14:03 | Walk-Run |
| 15 | | 1.5 | 20:25 | 13:37 | Walk-Run |
| 16 | | 1.5 | 19:48 | 13:12 | Walk-Run |

| Step | Max Mets | Distance (miles) | Target Time (min:sec) | Speed Minutes/Mile (min:sec) | Pace |
|------|----------|------------------|-----------------------|------------------------------|------|
| 17 | 9 | 2.5 | 34:07 | 13:38 | Walk-Run |
| 18 | | 2.0 | 26:22 | 13:11 | Walk-Run |
| 19 | | 1.5 | 19:08 | 12:45 | Walk-Run |
| 20 | | 1.5 | 18:32 | 12:21 | Walk-Run |
| 21 | 10 | 2.5 | 32:09 | 12:51 | Walk-Run |
| 22 | | 2.5 | 31:01 | 12:24 | Walk-Run |
| 23 | | 1.5 | 17:59 | 11:59 | Walk-Run |
| 24 | 11 | 2.5 | 30:21 | 12:08 | Walk-Run |
| 25 | | 1.5 | 17:33 | 11:42 | Walk-Run |
| 26 | | 1.5 | 16:56 | 11:17 | Run |
| 27 | 12 | 2.5 | 28:43 | 11:29 | Run |
| 28 | | 1.5 | 16:44 | 11:09 | Run |
| 29 | | 1.5 | 15:36 | 10:24 | Run |
| 30 | 13 | 2.5 | 27:04 | 10:49 | Run |
| 31 | | 1.5 | 15:05 | 10:03 | Run |
| 32 | | 2.0 | 18:46 | 9:23 | Run |
| 33 | | 2.5 | 22:01 | 8:48 | Run |
| 34 | | 2.5 | 20:43 | 8:17 | Run |
| 35 | 14 | 3.0 | 28:30 | 9:30 | Run |
| 36 | | 3.5 | 31:59 | 9:08 | Run |
| 37 | | 3.0 | 25:36 | 8:32 | Run |
| 38 | | 2.5 | 20:03 | 8:01 | Run |
| 39 | | 2.5 | 18:54 | 7:33 | Run |
| 40 | 15 | 3.5 | 31:23 | 8:58 | Run |
| 41 | | 3.5 | 29:15 | 8:21 | Run |
| 42 | | 3.0 | 23:27 | 7:49 | Run |
| 43 | | 2.5 | 18:23 | 7:21 | Run |
| 44 | 16 | 3.5 | 28:58 | 8:14 | Run |
| 45 | | 3.5 | 26:54 | 7:41 | Run |
| 46 | | 2.5 | 18:00 | 7:12 | Run |
| 47 | | 2.5 | 16:57 | 6:46 | Run |
| 48 | 17 | 3.5 | 26:37 | 7:36 | Run |
| 49 | | 4.0 | 28:24 | 7:06 | Run |
| 50 | | 2.5 | 16:40 | 6:40 | Run |
| 51 | | 3.5 | 21:58 | 6:16 | Run |

| Step | Max Mets | Distance (miles) | Target Time (min:sec) | Speed Minutes/Mile (min:sec) | Pace |
|------|----------|------------------|-----------------------|------------------------------|------|
| 52 | 18 | 4.5 | 31:43 | 7:03 | Run |
| 53 | | 4.0 | 26:20 | 6:35 | Run |
| 54 | | 3.5 | 21:41 | 6:11 | Run |
| 55 | | 3.5 | 20:26 | 5:50 | Run |
| 56 | 19 | 4.5 | 29:31 | 6:33 | Run |
| 57 | | 4.0 | 24:32 | 6:08 | Run |
| 58 | | 3.5 | 20:13 | 5:46 | Run |
| 59 | | 3.5 | 19:05 | 5:27 | Run |
| 60 | 20 | 4.5 | 27:34 | 6:07 | Run |
| 61 | | 4.5 | 25:48 | 5:44 | Run |
| 62 | | 3.5 | 18:55 | 5:24 | Run |
| 63 | 21 | 5.5 | 31:35 | 5:44 | Run |
| 64 | | 4.0 | 21:32 | 5:23 | Run |
| 65 | | 3.5 | 17:46 | 5:04 | Run |
| 66 | 22 | 5.5 | 29:40 | 5:23 | Run |
| 67 | | 4.5 | 22:48 | 5:04 | Run |

## "TOTAL JOCK" BICYCLE PROGRAM

Use three-mile bicycle test to determine your max mets. Start at your max met level. Remain at step until you can complete distance in target time.

| Step | Max Mets | Distance (miles) | Target Time (min:sec) | Speed (mph) |
|------|----------|------------------|-----------------------|-------------|
| 1 | 5 | 2.5 | 17:12 | 8.7 |
| 2 | | 3.0 | 19:54 | 9.0 |
| 3 | | 3.0 | 19:12 | 9.4 |
| 4 | | 3.5 | 21:39 | 9.7 |
| 5 | 6 | 4.0 | 24:53 | 9.6 |
| 6 | | 3.5 | 20:55 | 10.0 |
| 7 | | 3.5 | 20:08 | 10.4 |
| 8 | | 3.5 | 19:24 | 10.8 |
| 9 | 7 | 4.5 | 25:28 | 10.6 |
| 10 | | 3.5 | 18:59 | 11.1 |
| 11 | | 3.5 | 18:14 | 11.5 |
| 12 | | 3.5 | 17:32 | 12.0 |

| Step | Max Mets | Distance (miles) | Target Time (min:sec) | Speed (mph) |
|------|----------|------------------|-----------------------|-------------|
| 13 | 8 | 4.5 | 23:19 | 11.6 |
| 14 |   | 4.0 | 19:50 | 12.1 |
| 15 |   | 4.5 | 21:23 | 12.6 |
| 16 |   | 4.5 | 20:32 | 13.1 |
| 17 | 9 | 5.5 | 26:13 | 12.6 |
| 18 |   | 4.5 | 20:30 | 13.2 |
| 19 |   | 4.5 | 19:37 | 13.7 |
| 20 |   | 4.5 | 18:49 | 14.3 |
| 21 | 10 | 5.5 | 24:14 | 13.6 |
| 22 |   | 5.5 | 23:08 | 14.3 |
| 23 |   | 4.5 | 18:06 | 14.9 |
| 24 | 11 | 6.0 | 24:32 | 14.7 |
| 25 |   | 5.0 | 19:29 | 15.4 |
| 26 |   | 5.5 | 20:29 | 16.1 |
| 27 |   | 5.5 | 19:37 | 16.8 |
| 28 | 12 | 7.5 | 28:34 | 15.8 |
| 29 |   | 8.5 | 30:50 | 16.5 |
| 30 |   | 7.0 | 24:16 | 17.3 |
| 31 |   | 6.0 | 19:53 | 18.1 |
| 32 | 13 | 8.5 | 30:14 | 16.9 |
| 33 |   | 8.5 | 28:47 | 17.7 |
| 34 |   | 7.0 | 22:35 | 18.6 |
| 35 |   | 6.5 | 20:05 | 19.4 |
| 36 | 14 | 8.5 | 28:20 | 18.0 |
| 37 |   | 9.5 | 30:08 | 18.9 |
| 38 |   | 8.0 | 24:14 | 19.8 |
| 39 |   | 6.5 | 18:48 | 20.7 |
| 40 | 15 | 9.5 | 29:45 | 19.2 |
| 41 |   | 8.0 | 23:53 | 20.1 |
| 42 |   | 7.0 | 19:53 | 21.1 |
| 43 |   | 7.5 | 20:22 | 22.1 |
| 44 | 16 | 10.5 | 30:57 | 20.3 |
| 45 |   | 9.5 | 26:38 | 21.4 |
| 46 |   | 7.5 | 20:03 | 22.4 |
| 47 |   | 7.5 | 19:10 | 23.5 |

| Step | Max Mets | Distance (miles) | Target Time (min:sec) | Speed (mph) |
|------|----------|------------------|-----------------------|-------------|
| 48 | 17 | 10.5 | 29:13 | 21.5 |
| 49 | | 9.5 | 25:07 | 22.7 |
| 50 | | 7.5 | 18:55 | 23.7 |
| 51 | | 8.5 | 20:29 | 24.8 |
| 52 | 18 | 11.5 | 30:15 | 22.8 |
| 53 | | 10.5 | 26:15 | 24.0 |
| 54 | | 8.5 | 20:16 | 25.1 |
| 55 | | 8.5 | 19:22 | 26.3 |
| 56 | 19 | 12.0 | 29:55 | 24.9 |
| 57 | | 11.0 | 26:05 | 25.3 |
| 58 | | 8.5 | 19:12 | 26.5 |
| 59 | 20 | 12.5 | 29:34 | 25.4 |
| 60 | | 8.5 | 19:07 | 26.7 |
| 61 | | 9.5 | 20:22 | 28.0 |

## "TOTAL JOCK" SWIMMING PROGRAM

Use 400-yard swim test to determine your max mets. Start at the first step of your max met level. Remain at step until you can complete distance in target time.

| Step | Max Mets | Distance (yards) | Target Time (min:sec) |
|------|----------|------------------|-----------------------|
| 1 | 5 | 600 | 21:08 |
| 2 | | 600 | 20:35 |
| 3 | | 600 | 20:03 |
| 4 | | 600 | 19:34 |
| 5 | 6 | 700 | 22:55 |
| 6 | | 600 | 19:04 |
| 7 | | 600 | 18:32 |
| 8 | | 700 | 21:02 |

| Step | Max Mets | Distance (yards) | Target Time (min:sec) |
|------|----------|------------------|-----------------------|
| 9  | 7  | 800   | 24:25 |
| 10 |    | 700   | 20:41 |
| 11 |    | 700   | 20:03 |
| 12 |    | 700   | 19:28 |
| 13 |    | 700   | 18:54 |
| 14 | 8  | 800   | 22:49 |
| 15 |    | 800   | 22:03 |
| 16 |    | 700   | 18:40 |
| 17 |    | 800   | 20:40 |
| 18 |    | 800   | 20:02 |
| 19 | 9  | 850   | 22:44 |
| 20 |    | 950   | 24:38 |
| 21 |    | 800   | 19:56 |
| 22 |    | 800   | 19:16 |
| 23 |    | 900   | 20:59 |
| 24 | 10 | 1,000 | 25:08 |
| 25 |    | 1,000 | 24:12 |
| 26 |    | 1,100 | 25:41 |
| 27 |    | 1,100 | 24:48 |
| 28 |    | 1,100 | 23:58 |
| 29 | 11 | 1,300 | 30:46 |
| 30 |    | 1,300 | 29:35 |
| 31 |    | 1,300 | 28:30 |
| 32 |    | 1,200 | 25:23 |
| 33 |    | 1,200 | 24:31 |
| 34 | 12 | 1,400 | 31:32 |
| 35 |    | 1,400 | 30:02 |
| 36 |    | 1,400 | 28:54 |
| 37 |    | 1,300 | 25:52 |
| 38 |    | 1,300 | 24:57 |
| 39 | 13 | 1,500 | 32:03 |
| 40 |    | 1,400 | 28:22 |
| 41 |    | 1,500 | 29:13 |
| 42 |    | 1,300 | 24:23 |
| 43 |    | 1,400 | 25:19 |

| Step | Max Mets | Distance (yards ) | Target Time (min:sec) |
|------|----------|-------------------|-----------------------|
| 44   | 14       | 1,600             | 31:59                 |
| 45   |          | 1,600             | 30:41                 |
| 46   |          | 1,700             | 31:19                 |
| 47   |          | 1,400             | 24:49                 |
| 48   |          | 1,500             | 25:37                 |
| 49   | 15       | 1,600             | 30:21                 |
| 50   |          | 1,700             | 30:54                 |
| 51   |          | 1,700             | 29:40                 |
| 52   |          | 1,500             | 25:11                 |
| 53   | 16       | 1,800             | 32:36                 |
| 54   |          | 1,700             | 29:21                 |
| 55   |          | 1,500             | 24:51                 |
| 56   |          | 1,600             | 25:29                 |
| 57   | 17       | 1,800             | 30:52                 |
| 58   |          | 1,800             | 29:33                 |
| 59   |          | 1,600             | 25:12                 |
| 60   |          | 1,700             | 25:43                 |
| 61   | 18       | 1,800             | 29:24                 |
| 62   |          | 1,900             | 29:42                 |
| 63   |          | 1,700             | 25:29                 |
| 64   |          | 1,700             | 24:29                 |
| 65   | 19       | 1,900             | 29:37                 |
| 66   |          | 2,000             | 29:49                 |
| 67   |          | 1,700             | 24:18                 |
| 68   |          | 1,800             | 24:43                 |
| 69   | 20       | 2,100             | 30:02                 |
| 70   |          | 2,100             | 29:54                 |
| 71   |          | 1,800             | 24:34                 |
| 72   | 21       | 2,200             | 31:20                 |
| 73   |          | 1,800             | 24:30                 |
| 74   |          | 1,900             | 24:47                 |
| 75   | 22       | 2,100             | 28:37                 |
| 76   |          | 2,000             | 26:14                 |
| 77   |          | 2,000             | 24:58                 |

| Step | Max Mets | Distance (yards ) | Target Time (min:sec) |
|------|----------|-------------------|-----------------------|
| 78   | 23       | 2,200             | 28:44                 |
| 79   |          | 2,300             | 28:43                 |
| 80   |          | 2,100             | 25:07                 |
| 81   | 24       | 2,400             | 30:04                 |
| 82   |          | 2,400             | 28:45                 |

Sports and fitness are important at any age.

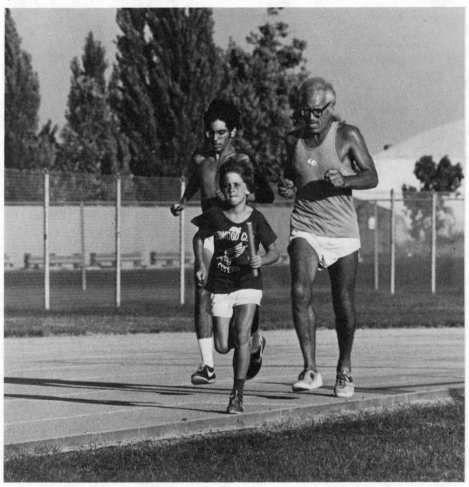

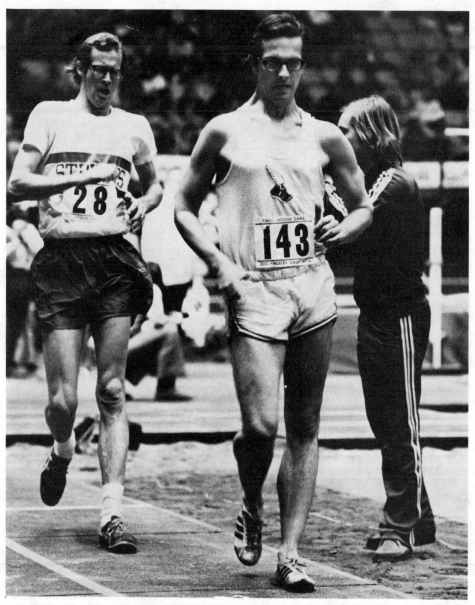

Race walking requires a high level of endurance.

## LONG, SLOW DISTANCE

Many people don't like to exercise by the clock. Although increasing the intensity of the workout is essential for improving your max mets, you can experience fitness increases by just running, swimming, and cycling for a long period of time. I personally enjoy going on an hour run. This type of training does affect your body's metabolism, particularly your ability to utilize fats. There is nothing wrong with this type of training. However, if you fail to work hard enough, you are not training as effectively as you could be. As a rule of thumb, you should be able to talk

A stationary bicycle is a good way to develop endurance when the weather is bad.

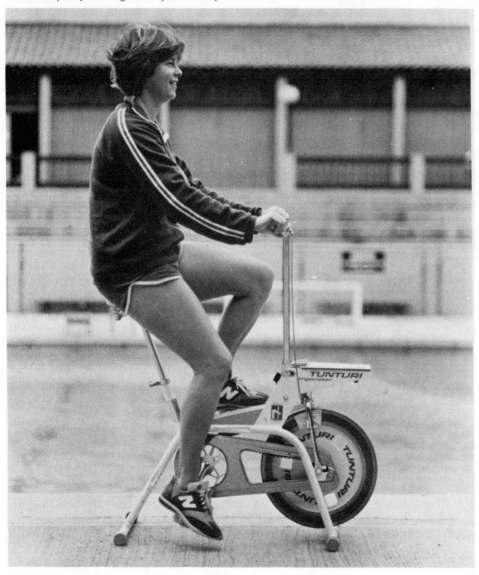

during your exercise (except swimming), but your heart rate should be at the target level (See Chapter 3 for your target heart rate).

Many people find running to a particular destination much easier than running around a track. I hate running laps around a track. I can't even remember the lap count on a three-mile run. I have a six-mile course I like to do. I run three miles to a reservoir. Once I get there, I have to come back. On that run I don't have to worry about mundane matters such as lap numbers; I can let my mind wander and enjoy the scenery.

Long, slow distance training has the advantage of allowing you to train in pleasant surroundings. It's nice to run in the park or out in the countryside without worrying about times and distances. Recently, during a snow drought in California, I spent two weeks at Christmastime running in the mountains. There were no people on the trail, and everyone in my group enjoyed themselves immensely. I wouldn't have used my computerized charts even if I had brought them.

The "Total Jock" exercise charts are designed to help you improve. If you never push yourself, you will not improve. Improvement requires you to regularly push your body a little harder than before.

There are many varieties of long, slow distance, such as Swedish fartlek training, which involves combining long, slow distance with periods of increased speed. This type of training can be applied to running, swimming, cycling, or cross-country skiing. You might go out and run a ten-minute mile pace. Then, for ¼ mile break into a rapid stride, followed by a 100-yard sprint. Then you would revert back to your ten-minute mile pace or walk for a while. Fartlek training is also called speed play. You basically mix up your training speed in a free sort of way. Do what you feel like.

## SKIING ON THE FLATS

Cross-country skiing is a great way to develop endurance. A friend of mine once told me, "If God wanted me to cross-country ski, he wouldn't have put ski lifts in the mountains." Personally, I prefer downhill skiing to almost any sport. However, downhill skiing has several severe drawbacks. Ski resorts are crowded. If you want to go up to the mountains to get away from people, forget about skiing. And downhill skiing is prohibitively expensive. A good complete ski outfit, including skis, boots, and clothes can cost over $500. When you add the cost of lifts, food, lodging, and drinks, you're talking about big bucks.

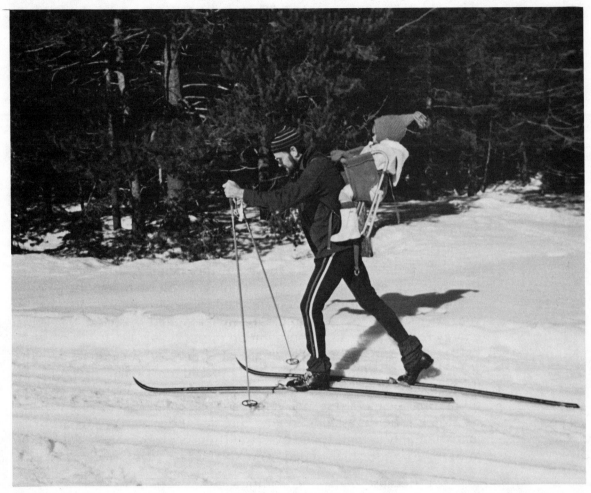

Cross-country skiing

Cross-country skiing is a good alternative. The equipment costs are less, and you can often go a whole day without seeing a soul. Because there are few restaurants and bars in the backwoods, you are forced to bring your own food and drink, which saves you money. Cross-country skiing is one of the best forms of endurance exercise. Although it's difficult to cross-country ski on a regular basis, it does provide an occasional alternative to running, swimming, or cycling. If you couple your cross-country skiing with camping, you can have a tremendous outdoor experience.

Related to cross-country skiing is ski touring. This involves not only skiing cross country, but going up and down mountains. One of my all-time great experiences was climbing Mt. Shasta in California and skiing down it. You can go down runs that may have never been skied before.

Ice skating can also provide good endurance exercise. In parts of Europe people can skate for miles, which definitely gives them the opportunity to use skating to improve endurance. In the United States few areas of the country provide this type of experience. Indoor ice rinks make it possible to a certain extent, but you have to work at it.

## QUICK AS A CAT: TRAINING FOR SPEED

Moving fast on a tennis court of down the bumps on a snowfield requires more than endurance training. You have to work out at high speeds to prepare yourself for these activities. Some sports scientists call this type of exercise anaerobic training because metabolic energy pathways not requiring oxygen are used to provide energy. In humans you always need oxygen, but during high speed exercise, anaerobic energy pathways become more important.

You have to be exceedingly careful before beginning a high-speed exercise program. You probably should have a max mets capacity of at least 13 before even thinking about this type of training. In addition to placing heavy stress on your cardiovascular system, high-speed training can be devastating to your muscles and joints. Your chances of injury multiply in high-speed exercise. These are some simple guidelines to prepare you for high-speed exercise.

1. Because high-speed running poses serious risk of injury, do not start this type of training until you are in shape.
2. Warm up thoroughly. This should include stretching and exercising at a slow rate. Gradually increase the pace of your warm-up until you are reaching the full speed of your workout.
3. Don't practice this type of training more than two days a week. Too much high-speed training may lead to chronic fatigue and increased risk of injury.
4. Don't do too much too soon. Overdoing this type of exercise may result in muscle soreness that won't subside for a week.

There are many kinds of high-speed training. You can increase your body's capacity for rapid exercise by playing high-intensity sports such as basketball, racquetball, and badminton. Probably the best way of developing this capacity is interval training—repeatedly exercising at relatively short distances. Exercises such as rope skipping and the "Total Jock" speed program will also improve your ability to perform high-intensity exercise.

## Interval Training

Interval training is used by coaches throughout the world in many sports to improve high-speed fitness. You can use interval training for exercises such as running, swimming, and cycling. Interval training involves manipulating factors of training for the purpose of improving speed. These factors are

1. Distance
2. Speed
3. Repetitions
4. Rest intervals between repetitions

An example of interval training for running would be

1. Distance: 440 yards
2. Speed: 80 to 90 seconds
3. Repetitions: four
4. Rest interval between repetitions: five minutes

This means you run 440 yards four times with a five-minute rest period between runs. Each 440-yard run should be done in 80 to 90 seconds. Interval training is a great way to improve your fitness for high-intensity sports. The principles of interval training are the same for cycling, swimming, and running. You can literally figure out thousands of combinations for this type of exercise. In general, the faster the speed of the interval, the fewer the number of repetitions and the longer the rest period between intervals. I have provided several examples of intervals. Experiment with many programs and choose the one best suited to you.

Example 1:
*Short Sprint Interval Training*
1. Type of exercise: sprint running on 440-yard track; sprint straightaways, walk turns
2. Distance: 100-yard sprints

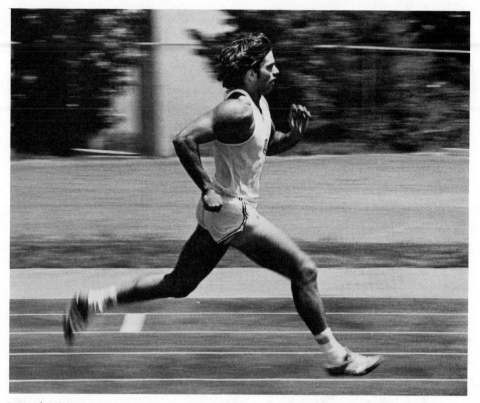
Interval training

3. Speed: 8/10 of your full speed
4. Repetitions: eight (total of one mile with sprints and walking)
5. Rest period: time it takes to walk turn, approximately three minutes between each sprint.

*Swimming Intervals*
1. Type of exercise: swimming, medium distance
2. Distance: 100 yards
3. Speed: full speed
4. Repetitions: five to ten
5. Rest period: three to five minutes

*Middle Distance Running*
1. Type of exercise: middle distance running
2. Distance: 880 yards

3. Speed: best 880 time plus 30 seconds
4. Repetitions: four
5. Rest period: five minutes

I want to emphasize that you must not overdo this type of training. Your muscles and liver have a maximum storage capacity for glycogen of about 250 grams. Glycogen, as you remember, is the most important fuel for muscular work. During heavy exercise, you use up your glycogen at a rapid rate. It takes time to rebuild your glycogen stores. If you overdo this type of training, you may be letting yourself in for chronic fatigue.

## ROPE SKIPPING

I learned how to skip rope by watching ex-heavyweight boxing champion Sonny Liston training to the tune of "Night Train." His preparations for a fight in Las Vegas were shown on TV. By watching him, I was able to pick up the intricate rhythm of this type of exercise. Rope skipping is a good way to develop a metabolism adapted to high-speed exercise.

There are many variations you can learn that will increase your fitness and at the same time impress your friends with your athletic skill. Start off by bouncing on the ground twice for each revolution of the rope. Then bounce only once. After you've mastered the basics, try alternating your feet. Pretty soon you will be ready for the razzle-dazzle stuff—crossing your hands and completing two or three revolutions of the rope for one bounce.

You can arrange your rope skipping routine in a manner similar to interval training. For example

1. Time: 1 minute, alternating feet
2. Repetitions: ten
3. Rest between repetitions: one minute

If you are serious about rope skipping, buy a good rope. Ideally, purchase a leather rope with wooden handles. The handle should contain bearings to help the rope rotate easily. Although rope skipping is a good exercise, it should not be used as a substitute for endurance exercise unless you can jump continuously for at least 15 to 20 minutes. Remember, your body's metabolism reacts differently to short-term, high-intensity exercise and lower-intensity endurance training.

# INCREASING YOUR RUNNING SPEED

Sprint speed seems to be genetically determined to a large extent. If you can run only a 14-second 100-yard dash, you had better forget about the world record. However, you can improve your speed somewhat. Two factors determine sprint speed:

1. Length of stride
2. Frequency of stride

By increasing these factors, you can improve your speed. There is a delicate balance between stride frequency and stride length. If your stride length is too long, your stride frequency will decrease. If you try to increase your frequency, your stride length may decrease. The only way you can increase your speed is to increase your ability to exert force at fast speeds of motion.

# THE "TOTAL JOCK" SPEED PROGRAM

The "Total Jock" speed program uses a variety of techniques to increase sprinting capacity:

1. High knee exercise
2. Long stride exercise
3. Downhill sprinting
4. The harness
5. Isokinetic bicycle

With the exception of the isokinetic bicycle, all these techniques are readily available and will help you improve your speed.

## High Knee Exercise

This exercise involves lifting the knees high very rapidly and pumping the arms in an exaggerated sprinting motion. You should take at least ten strides for every ten yards. The majority of world-class sprinters practice this exercise. An example of training routine would be to practice this for five repetitions of 50 yards.

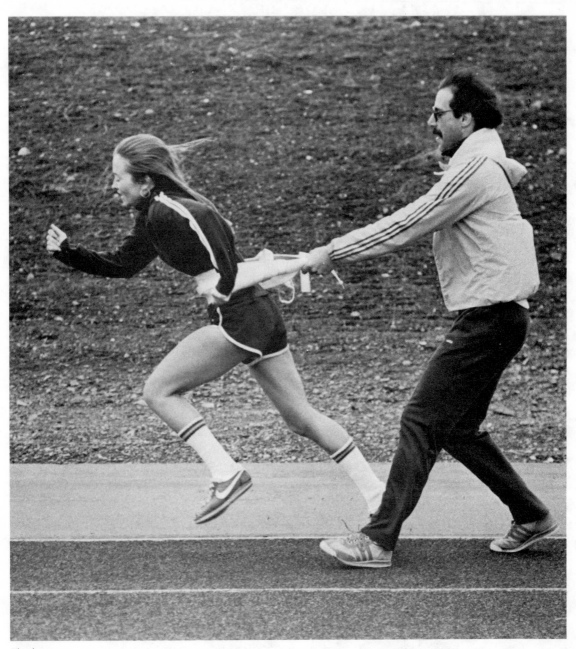

The harness

## Long Stride Exercise

For this exercise you run a distance of 100 yards, taking as few strides as possible. This involves a series of bounding leaps. A training example would be five repetitions of 100 yards.

## Downhill Sprinting

This is a new technique that's been used by several successful sprinters. By sprinting downhill, you train your body to increase its stride frequency. Find a hill with a small decline at first, then graduate to something steeper. Be careful about the surface you run on. This type of training may result in injury if you're not careful.

## The Harness

The harness allows you to run against resistance and thus increase your strength. Tape a towel on a rope and then put the towel at waist level. Have someone hold the rope and provide resistance as you run. Try to exaggerate the high knee action and rapid pumping of the arms.

An example of a harness workout would be to run five repetitions of 50 yards.

## Isokinetic Bicycle

An isokinetic exercise involves exerting force at a constant speed. This is an artificial type of movement possible only on isokinetic exercise machines. These machines are designed to help you increase your strength at fast speeds of movement.

Isokinetic bicycles help you to increase your stride frequency. Your training regime consists of gradually increasing your pedal revolutions as you get faster. This type of bicycle is available in health clubs and at several universities in their physical education program.

## DEVELOPING QUICKNESS FOR SPORTS

Sports skills are extremely specific. You can best improve your efficiency by endless practice. Learn to make your movements as simple as possible. Unnecessary motion slows you down and decreases your effectiveness. Learn the fundamentals of footwork and body position early and avoid developing bad habits that will plague you. By maximizing your fitness, mastering fundamentals, and practicing your skills, you can be quicker and more graceful.

There are many drills that develop specific sports skills. Drills should closely approximate the skills actually used in a sport. Your drills should be practiced at about the same speed as the actual activity. Avoid general drills that promise to develop quick feet. Football grass drills, in which you change your body position rapidly, may aid in physical conditioning, but they do little to improve the quickness required in a specific sport. Practice should reflect the requirements of the sports as closely as possible.

## INSTANT REPLAY

1. You must practice endurance exercise to improve your max mets. Use the computerized exercise programs for running, bicycling, and swimming to progress at the fastest possible rate.
2. You should practice endurance exercise three to five days per week.
3. Don't do high-speed training more than two days a week.
4. Speed exercises are important for developing the fitness required in many sports.

# CHAP 8 TER

# STRENGTH AND POWER FOR SPORTS

In my youth I sat on the edge of my chair at the movies as Steve Reeves, playing the role of Hercules, threw a discus out of the stadium, a distance of at least three miles (a world record). Reeves, formerly Mr. America, did much to popularize strength training. His successor in the public eye, Arnold Schwarzenegger, has made weight training and body building almost respectable. Ten years ago a woman would have been considered highly eccentric if she ventured into the almost totally male domiciles where weights were lifted. Now there are women's weight training classes, and coeducational exercise areas are commonplace.

Strength training has been recognized as almost essential for improving the strength and power required in sports. More strength allows you to move more forcefully. You can hit a tennis ball harder, and you can maintain a correct position in skiing for a longer time. Strength is an area of fitness neglected by many. With a relatively small time commitment, you can add power to your movements and at the same time develop a more attractive body.

Endurance and flexibility exercises alone will not give you a nice body. Strength training provides you with a firmer, more shapely physique. For women this means a sleek, attractive body. For men this means larger, more shapely muscles. Strength exercises will give you more sex appeal. Just as important, these exercises will improve your sports performances. When you're stronger, you will be playing at a lower percentage of your maximum strength. You will fatigue less easily.

Strength training is part of the programs of athletes ranging from distance runners to football players. If you want to get better at sports, then you'd better do some of these exercises regularly. There are many varieties of strength training programs. If you learn the correct principles, you can choose the method that's right for you.

# STRENGTH AND ENDURANCE FITNESS

Athletic equipment manufacturers sometimes try to get you to believe their product will do all things for your fitness program. They are much like snake oil salesmen who claim their mixture will do everything from curing cancer to removing warts. Strength plays an important role in fitness, but it is by no means the only factor. Beware of health club "experts" who tell you their exercise machines will develop significant cardiovascular endurance while maximizing strength gains. Your body reacts to the stresses placed upon it. If you stress your body's cardiovascular endurance, then that component of fitness improves. No one type of exercise is a magic panacea for total fitness. Forget about that gadget you can fit in a desk drawer that gives you fitness in five minutes a day. It's just more junk to clutter up your house.

Heart rate is a valid measure of cardiovascular conditioning only when the exercise is continuous, rhythmic, and uses large muscle areas. Although short-term, high-intensity exercises such as weight training may raise the heart rate to very high levels, they are of little value in promoting cardiovascular endurance. Remember, it takes several minutes of continuous exercise to redistribute blood (and thus oxygen) to your working muscles. Research studies have shown that strength exercises use muscle fibers that do not require as much oxygen for supplying their energy needs. Cardiovascular conditioning partially depends on the development of the endurance muscle fibers (slow twitch fibers). These fibers are not used to a great extent in weight training exercise.

The work of the heart has been studied during different types of exercise with a procedure called echocardiography. Weight training exercise affects the heart much differently than endurance training. Strength training raises your heart rate and blood pressure because of a reflex called the valsava phenomenon. When you strain to lift a weight, you raise the pressure within your chest cavity, which causes your heart to beat faster. So, although your heart may beat rapidly, you receive little cardiovascular conditioning. Heart rate is a valuable measure of endurance training when it reflects the stress on your metabolism. Watching scary movies may raise your heart rate, but it cannot be considered endurance exercise.

Strength training may help your endurance performance, but it should not replace it. Don't be fooled by training devices that promise total fitness. Many of these devices do improve certain aspects of your fitness and are therefore valuable. However, none will make you totally fit. It just isn't that easy.

## Specificity of Strength

There is a specificity of strength. I have known people who could bench press (lift barbell off the chest from a bench) over 400 pounds and yet were incapable of using this strength. Many athletes spend a lot of time developing strength in the weight room and neglect their athletic skills. You have to incorporate strength increases into your sports technique or it's useless.

Recently, we conducted an exercise training study with teenage girls and boys. Their training program included heavy weight training during an eight-week period. We found large increases in their strength. However, when we tested their ability to exert their new strength at fast speeds of movement, their improvements were less impressive. You have to develop strength in a way that is useful to your athletic performance. The strength program for the shot-putter is different from that of the runner. A person with well-rounded fitness needs a balanced strength program.

## Types of Strength

Strength manifests itself differently in various activities. The golfer needs a controlled application of force at the right time, while the skier has to maintain a moderate level of strength throughout the day. There are really different kinds of strengths. Train your body for the strength needed for your sports. For the jock this should be well-rounded strength that prepares you for a variety of activities.

There are three basic categories of strength:

1. Maximum force
2. Power
3. Sustained force (strength-endurance)

Maximum force is the ability to exhibit brute strength. Lifting heavy weights, opening up sticky jelly jars, or prying a rock from the ground are examples. This is probably the factor most emphasized by strength trainers.

When I was a discus thrower, I also dabbled in competitive

weight lifting (power lifting). I spent countless hours trying to develop my bench press, squat, and dead lift. Although I think picking up huge barbells has intrinsic value (ego, big muscles), you must analyze the value of such a program. If your goal is to bench press 400 pounds, then by all means continue. However, if your goal is to improve at sports, you should carefully consider the type of strength exercises and the muscles you are building.

In general, try to strengthen your muscles in a manner similar to their use in sports. If legs are important in a sport, work on your legs. This sounds obvious, but many athletes ignore this simple principle. For example, in a sport like football, the legs are of primary importance for performance and preventing injury. The majority of college football players and even a few pros have tremendously strong upper bodies, but they often have bird-like lower bodies. Some athletes who can bench press over 400 pounds are incapable of doing squats (knee bends) with 200 pounds.

Power is the most important strength characteristic of most sports. Power is the ability to exert force rapidly. Pushing big weights off your chest is of little value unless you can translate this into power. When an opponent rifles a serve that you can hardly see, let alone hit,

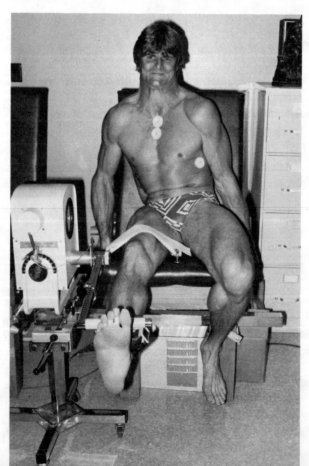

Brian Oldfield, world record holder in shotput, being tested on the Cybex.

you can bet there is effective power behind it. Power is something anyone can improve. You can often make up for undeveloped technique if you have good power. When you put power and technique together, you'll be dynamite. This combination is exhibited by many members of the Japanese women's volleyball team. They not only possess breathtaking skills but can muster awesome power in their shots. Bryan Oldfield, the world record holder in the shotput, is one of the most explosive athletes I have measured in my laboratory. He was so powerful he exceeded the capacity of one of my strength measuring instruments (Cybex II). At one time he combined a fluid technique with superior power to lead the world in the shotput by an incredible five feet.

Strength endurance, the third category, is the ability to maintain a level of strength for a sustained period of time. This type of strength is important for sports such as running, skiing, mountain climbing, and cycling. Your muscles react to a program of high repetition strength exercises by increasing their strength endurance. Researchers at Stanford have found that even heart patients can lessen the strain of exercise if they increase their strength endurance.

## TYPES OF STRENGTH TRAINING METHODS

Strength training methods have one thing in common: They all overload the muscles to do more than they have done in the past. Exercise regimens can be divided into four basic categories:

1. Isometric
2. Constant resistance
3. Variable resistance
4. Constant speed (isokinetic)

Isometric exercise is exerting force against an immovable object. This could be something like pushing against a wall or pitting one of your body parts against another. This type of exercise was made popular in the late 1950's because of the research of two German scientists, Hettinger and Mueller. They used isometrics with hospital patients and had great success. As often happens with scientific research, the findings were generalized to the healthy population and to athletes. Although isometrics develop a type of strength, they are of little use for sports. They do not develop the ability for more forceful movements and may even cause serious muscle injury.

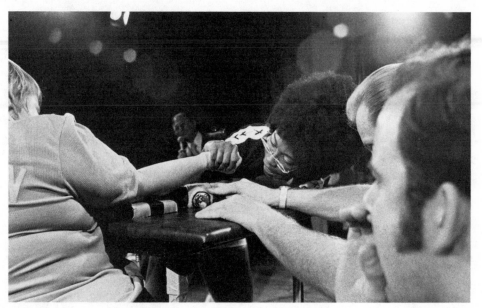

Arm wrestling is partially isometric.

You are probably most familiar with constant resistance exercise. In this type of training you attempt to move a weight against gravity. The resistance could be a barbell or dumbbell, or it could be your own body weight. So, when you do pushups or chinups, you are really weight training. Constant resistance is the most popular form of strength training for athletes and body builders. There are several advantages of this type of strength training:

1. Weight equipment is readily available. Practically every high school, college, and health club has this type of equipment. You can even purchase a barbell set for your home at a modest cost.
2. When you use your body weight as a resistance, you have even more flexibility. You can do simple arm and leg strengthening exercises anywhere.
3. The effectiveness of this type of training has been thoroughly demonstrated over the past 20 years. Training programs are well known and readily available.

Constant resistance exercise has several disadvantages:

1. The training effect is not constant throughout the muscle. When you move a weight against gravity, it's easier at some

points and more difficult at others. You do not develop strength at a uniform rate throughout the range of motion.

2. Strength is not developed as effectively at faster speeds of motion. Because you are training at relatively slow speeds, you gain strength for movements more slowly than those commonly required in sports.

3. This type of training seems to cause more severe muscle soreness.

You can adapt your strength training to your needs. Strength endurance, for example, is best developed by performing a relatively high number of repetitions (usually 10 to 15). To gain more strength and power, you should do fewer repetitions, which should allow you to use more weight. By moving the weight as rapidly as possible, you develop a type of strength more specific to sports.

Variable resistance training is relatively new and provides formerly unavailable ways of gaining strength. Variable resistance employs

Lahsen Akka, two-time Olympian, doing a power clean.

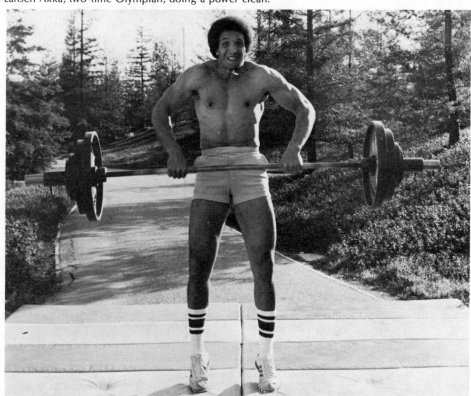

exercise machines, such as those manufactured by Nautilus and Universal Gym, that cause a uniform resistance throughout a range of motion. They make a movement tough to perform throughout the entire exercise. The manufacturers of these devices have developed special training regimens to accompany their machines. Nautilus, for example, has a number of machines that develop very specific muscle groups. They advise that the exercises be performed very slowly and with a high number of repetitions. Nautilus training is good for developing strength endurance as well as muscle flexibility, which is sometimes impaired by other types of strength training methods.

Constant speed exercise is also called isokinetic exercise. I think this type of training is the most significant exercise development since the advent of weight training. These exercise devices allow you to develop strength at fast speeds of motion. The result will be strength you can use in sports. Strength training is most effective when it is practiced at speeds used in sports. At present, these devices are not readily available, but I'm sure this situation will change as their worth is recognized. Isokinetic training requires tremendous concentration to be effective. You have to go full blast to get the full benefit. It's possible to perform the exercises and yet expend less than maximum effort.

## Strength Exercises Without Equipment

There are many exercises you can do that will develop your strength but require nothing other than your own body. Build up to the recommended sets and repetitions. Start off with one set and then gradually increase the severity of your workout. You don't need to do all of the exercises listed. Choose two or three from each category. Practice these exercises three days a week.

### EXERCISES FOR THE LEGS

1. Phantom Chair: This is great for skiers. Assume a seated position up against a wall. Keep feet flat on the floor and align your thighs parallel to the ground. Extend your arms in front of you. This exercise is a killer. Start by holding this position for 15 to 30 seconds. Gradually increase the time until you can go three minutes. Do one to three sets.

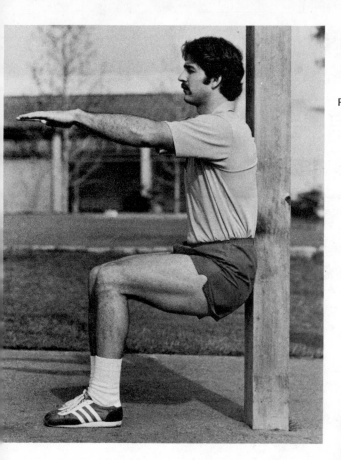

Phantom chair

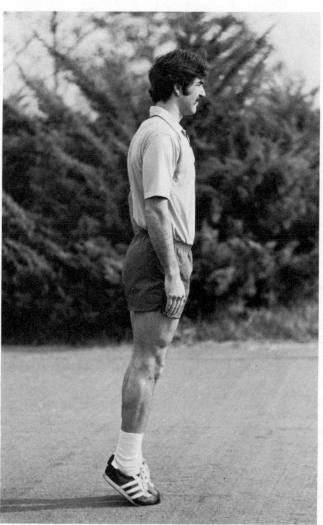

Toe raisers

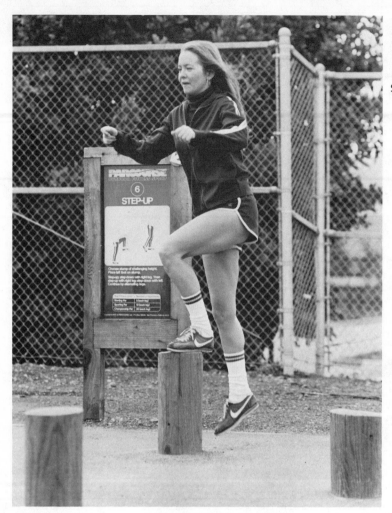

Step ups

Running stairs

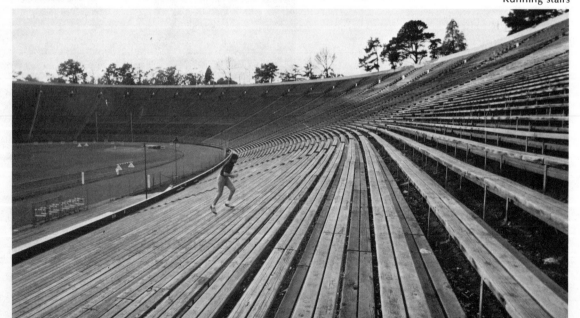

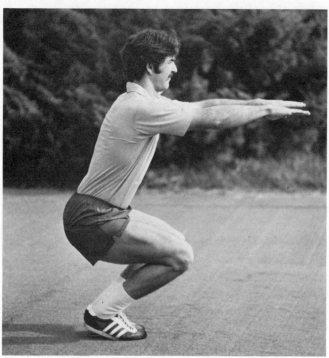
Knee bends

2. Step Ups: Step up on a bench or chair. Do ten repetitions with the left leg and then do ten repetitions with the right leg. Do three sets of this exercise.

3. Knee Bends: With feet approximately shoulder width apart, bend your knees until your thighs are parallel to the ground. Do three sets of ten repetitions. As an alternate, do this exercise very slowly. Go down gradually to a count of five, and then gradually return to a standing position.

4. Stair Climbing: Find a high school or college football stadium. Run up the steps. Start off slowly. Be careful on the way down. Don't do this exercise until you are in good shape. If you have knee trouble, check with your physician before doing this one; stair climbing may be hazardous to your knees. The number of repetitions and sets will depend upon the size of the stadium. A 100,000-seat stadium can have a lot of stairs.

5. Toe Raisers: From a standing position, lift your heels off the ground, and go up on your toes. Return to starting position. Do three sets of 10 to 20 repetitions.

6. Shins: Put feet under a low bar (four inches off ground) or under a fence. You can also have someone hold down your toes. Attempt to pull your toes upward toward your shins and

hold for a count of 10 to 20. Do three sets of this exercise. This is a good exercise to prevent shin splints (pains in front of your legs).

## ABDOMINAL AND BACK EXERCISES

1. Bent Knee Situps: Lie on your back; bend your knees and put your feet flat on the floor. Put your hands behind your head. Bend at the waist and touch your elbows to your knees. If you have trouble with this one, fold your arms across your chest rather than putting your hands behind your head. It's very important to keep your knees bent. Bent knees will prevent back strain and will exercise your abdominal muscles more thoroughly. Start with one set of ten repetitions. Build up to about two to three sets of 50 repetitions.
2. Twists: Put a broom handle on your shoulders and grasp it with both hands. Rotate from one side to the other. Do three sets of 25 to 50 repetitions.
3. Side Bends: From a standing position with arms at your sides, bend to one side and then to the other. Do three sets of 25 to 50 repetitions.

Situps

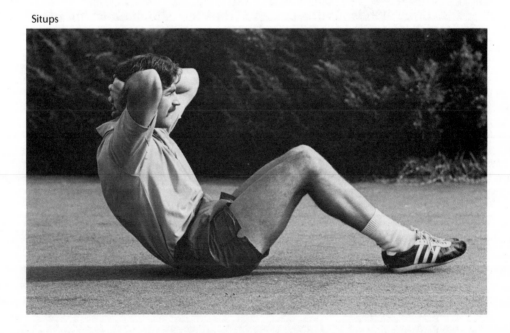

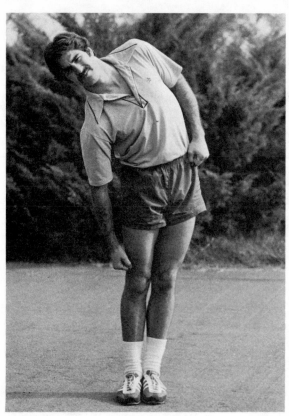

Side bends

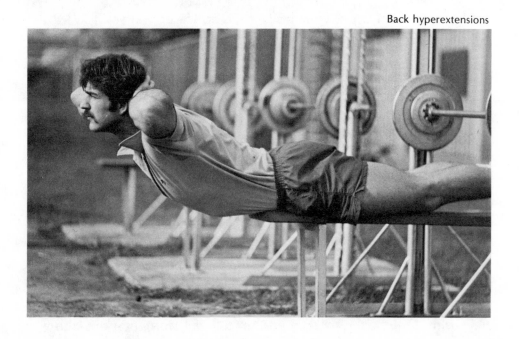

Back hyperextensions

4. Back Hyperextensions: Lie face down on a table with your upper body suspended unsupported over the edge. Have someone sit on your legs. Bend downward at the waist, and then return to the starting position. This is a great exercise for back strength. If you have back trouble, check with your doctor before doing this exercise. Build up to three sets of ten repetitions. You may want to begin by arching from the floor and then progressing to the floor.

## UPPER BODY EXERCISES

1. Pullups (chinups): Find a pullup bar. They are usually located in a school yard, or you can purchase one that will fit in a doorway. When I was a kid, I used a gas pipe until it broke and almost caused our house to burn down. Hang from the bar and attempt to pull yourself up. Your palms can either be facing toward you or away from you. Most people have a lot of trouble with this exercise. If you can't do a pullup, hang from the bar for three sets of ten seconds. Keep working on this, and you will eventually be successful. Build up to three sets of ten repetitions.
2. Pushups: The old standby. Support yourself on your hands and toes. Keeping your body straight, lower yourself toward the ground until your chest touches, then push yourself up. Make sure your back and stomach are stabilized. Pushups can be modified by supporting yourself on your knees instead of your toes. Build up to three sets of 20 repetitions.
3. Chair Dips: Put two solid chairs about shoulder width apart. Facing upward, support yourself by placing a hand on each chair and your heels on the ground with your legs stretched out. Lower yourself between the two chairs and then push yourself back to the starting position. Be careful that the chairs don't fall over.

## Pumping Iron

I spent much of my time in college at the Sunset Weight Lifting Club in San Francisco. Although the gym was far from being a showplace, it was extremely well equipped and had enough weights for Atlas himself to train with. One of the most important things I learned at the club was

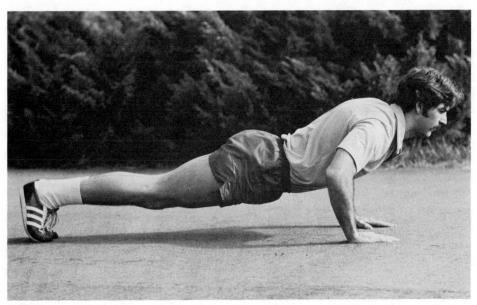
Pushups

that developing superior strength required training with strong people and demanded tremendous dedication. You just can't develop the necessary psyche needed for success by training in your back bedroom. To get strong you have to train at a gym.

Health clubs range from hard core weight lifting gyms to fancy, carpeted facilities complete with whirlpool baths, chrome equipment, and social director. A serious jock should join some kind of club. Strength is extremely important for sports. A health club membership will help you develop that strength. Shop around. Don't get swindled into joining a club for 20 years. Health clubs make their money from members who won't use the facilities. Start off with a limited membership. If you like the club, then sign up for a longer period of time. Beware of advice received from "health club experts." Most of these people are untrained and misinformed. Learn the correct principles of training and make your own decisions.

## PRINCIPLES OF WEIGHT TRAINING

1. Increased strength comes about by consistently working a little harder than before. This is the overload principle. If you don't push yourself consistently, you can't expect to improve.

2. Generally speaking, you should do a high number of repetitions (10 to 15) to increase strength endurance. If you are trying to improve your strength for endurance exercise, such as running or cycling, then do a lot of repetitions.
3. To improve the ability to exert a lot of force all at once, do fewer repetitions (one to five) and use more weight.
4. Body builders generally do many sets and many repetitions of an exercise. Top body builders spend as much as six hours a day in the gym.
5. Effective strength training requires ridding yourself of inhibitions. You have got to let it all hang out to get the best results. Some people go to great extremes to accomplish this. One guy at the Sunset gym was the first teenager in California to bench press 400 pounds. He would regularly run through Golden Gate Park growling like an animal to minimize his inhibitions. That's pretty bizarre behavior. Maybe you could try it in the privacy of your house before doing it in public.
6. Women don't develop large muscles from weight training. Typically, women lose fat and gain some muscle from strength exercises. Male hormones are required for large muscle development, so women increase their muscle size much more slowly. This type of training will develop a considerable amount of strength in women, which is important for sports. Many women ignore this important fitness component.
7. It's best to train three days per week. Pick specific days of the week, and stick to them. Monday, Wednesday, and Friday are favored by many. Two days a week is the minimum amount of time you can expect to strength train and still receive benefit.
8. A strength program designed to develop maximum power for sports should contain three components: a shoulder press (bench press, military press, incline press), a pulling exercise (clean, snatch, high pull), and a leg pressing exercise (squats, leg press). These exercises will be described.
9. Do your large muscle exercises first. For example, doing exercises for the wrists or biceps first will hamper your strength gains in shoulder and chest exercises.
10. Hustle through your workout. It's easy to get involved in gym chatter and not get any work done. Unless you really get into strength training, your workout should not exceed 1½ hours.
11. Warm up before pushing hard. Perform the exercise with a weight you can do easily before really going for it.

12. Well-rounded strength requires a variety of exercises to develop many areas of your body. When I was in high school, there was a guy who didn't follow this principle. He owned a souped-up 1957 Chevy with flames adorning the paint job on the fins of the car. He took great pleasure in cruising the local high school hangouts. He would circle the block hundreds of times with his left arm perched on the edge of his rolled down window. To magnify his stud image, he regularly practiced concentrated barbell curls with his left arm. The result was a massive Popeye-like development on his left side. The rest of his body was a bit withered. To the world outside his car he looked huge, with his cigarettes rolled up in his T-shirt sleeve and a tattoo of an anchor embossed on his muscular upper arm. But when he stepped out of his Chevy, he looked pretty ridiculous.

## Weight Training Exercises

When beginning a weight training program, select a weight for each exercise that you can do easily for ten repetitions. For the first workout do only one set. Then gradually increase until you build up to three sets. There are countless exercises that you can do and numerous program variations. I will show you some of the more common exercises you can do with a barbell set at home. I will also provide a sample workout schedule. I suggest you experiment and develop a program satisfying to you.

**LEG EXERCISES:**

1. Squats: Put a barbell on your shoulders with legs a comfortable distance apart. You might try putting a board under your heels to help your balance. Bend your knees until your thighs are parallel with the ground. Keep your head up, and try to do this exercise with your legs rather than your back. Go down slowly and up quickly. Have someone watch you do the exercise (spotter) so that he can help you if you encounter difficulty. Emphasize good technique to avoid injuring your back.
2. Toe Raisers: Same as the exercise described in the non-equipment exercises. Place barbell on your shoulders and rise

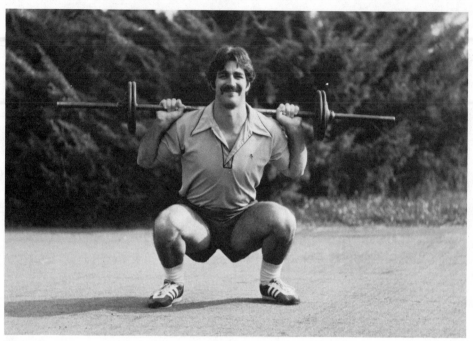

Squats

up on your toes. A good time to do this exercise is immediately after your squats.

## PULLING EXERCISES

1. Cleans: Stand with feet under the bar. Place your hands on the bar at about shoulder width. Keep your head up and your arms straight. The lift involves two pulling actions that are blended together in a flowing motion. The first pull brings the bar just below the knees, using mostly the legs and raising the head. The second pull involves driving the hips forward and arching the back. You go up on your toes and pull the weight up to your chest, supporting the weight with your hands. Try to watch your technique on every repetition to prevent injury. Variations of this exercise are the high pull and the snatch. The high pull is the same as the clean except that the weight is not supported at the chest. You just pull the weight as high as you can and retirn the weight to the floor. A description of the snatch is beyond the scope of this book. The snatch involves

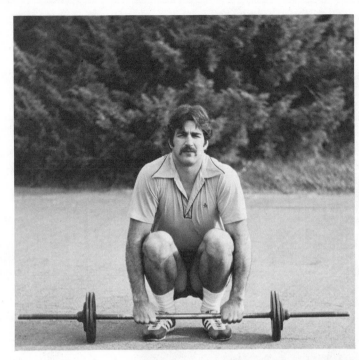

Sequence 1

The clean

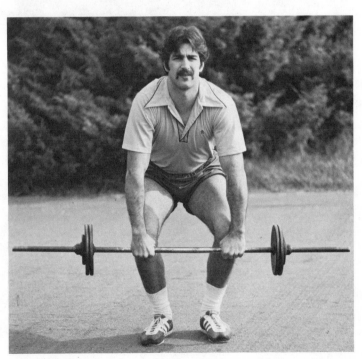

Sequence 2

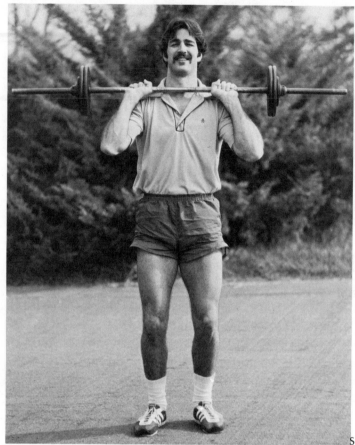

Sequence 3

pulling a barbell over your head in one continuous motion. The movement is extremely complex. If you want to learn the snatch, see a knowledgeable weight lifting coach or weight lifter.

## PRESSES

There are many varieties of shoulder presses. These exercises develop primarily the shoulders, arms, and chest.

1. Bench Press: This is a favorite exercise with most weight trainers. For women this exercise is valuable for firming the

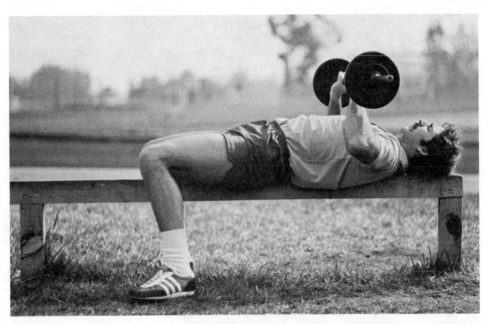

Bench press

bustline because of the effect on the muscles of the chest. You need a good solid bench with supports to put the barbell on. Lie down on the bench on your back. Keep your feet flat on the floor and start with the bar over your chest. Lower the weight until it touches your chest, then press the weight back to the starting position. There are many alternatives and variations to the bench press. Dumbbell bench presses are popular, especially with body builders. Incline presses are executed with either barbells or dumbbells. An incline press is done on a bench slanted at a 45-degree angle.

2. Shoulder Press: Shoulder presses are similar to bench presses except that the weights are pushed over the head. Standing presses are potentially dangerous to the back. If you do this type of exercise, it's best to sit on a bench so that your back gets some measure of support. These exercises can be accomplished with dumbbells and barbells. A competitive weight

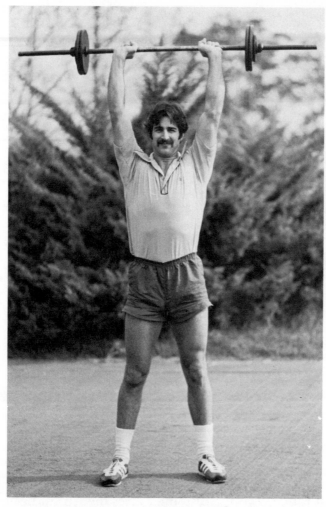

Shoulder press

lifting variation is the jerk, where a barbell is explosively pushed overhead.

## ARM EXERCISES

1. Biceps Curls: Grasp a bar with palms facing upward. Start with arms extended. Bend your elbows until the bar touches your chest. This exercise can be done with dumbbells and barbells. There are special curl bars that have bends in the shaft and are designed to lessen the strain on your forearm muscles.

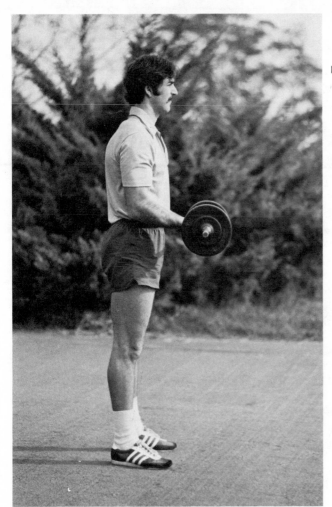

Biceps curls

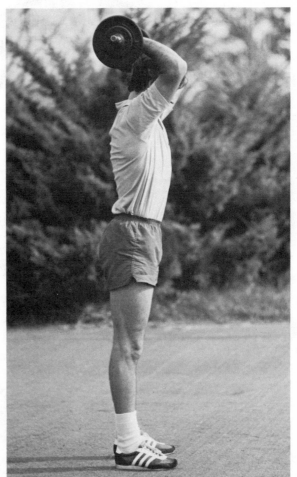

French curls

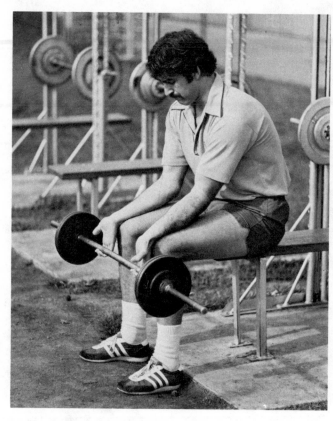

Wrist curls

2. French Curls: In a standing position, hold a barbell behind
   your neck with a narrow grip and elbows pointed upward.
   Extend your arms until your elbows are straight, and then
   slowly return to the starting position.
3. Wrist Curls: Sit on a chair with your forearms resting on your
   thighs and your wrists lying over your kneecaps, palms facing
   upward. Hold a bar in both hands and let your hands bend
   backward. Bend your wrists upward, and then return to
   starting position. This exercise can also be done with the palms
   facing downward.

## BACK EXERCISES

1. Pullovers: This exercise works muscles in your upper and
   middle back as well as in your shoulders and arms. Lie on a

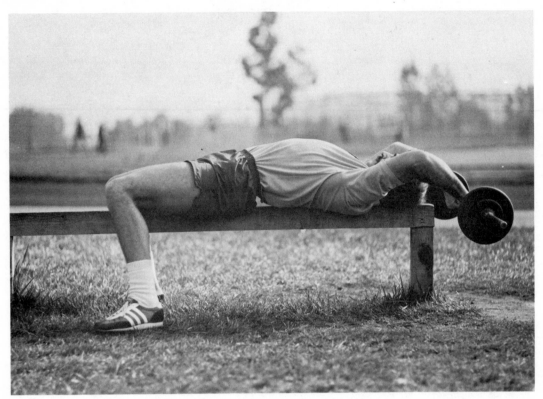
Pullovers

bench on your back with a barbell in both of your hands on
your chest. Lower the weight behind your head and below the
top of the bench. Pull the weight back to the starting position.
2. Good Morning Exercise: Put a light barbell on your shoulders.
From a standing position, bend your knees slightly. Keep your
head up and bend forward at your waist. Be careful with this
one. It's good to be overly conservative with the amount of
weight. Progress gradually.

## Sample Weight Programs

There are many types of weight programs. When you get into it, you will
discover the type of program that's best for you. Here are a few examples
for people with different amounts of experience.

## BEGINNER PROGRAM
Monday-Wednesday-Friday

| Exercise | Sets | Repetitions |
|---|---|---|
| Bench Press | 1–3 | 10 |
| Cleans | 1–3 | 5–10 |
| Squats | 1–3 | 5–10 |
| Biceps Curls | 1–3 | 10 |
| French Curls | 1–3 | 10 |
| Pullovers | 1–3 | 10 |
| Situps | 1–3 | 25 |

## INTERMEDIATE PROGRAM
Monday-Wednesday-Friday

| Exercise | Sets | Repetitions |
|---|---|---|
| Bench Press | 5 | 5 |
| Cleans | 5 | 5 |
| Squats | 5 | 5 |
| Biceps Curls | 3 | 10 |
| French Curls | 3 | 10 |
| Pullovers | 3 | 10 |
| Situps | 3 | 25 |

## ADVANCED PROGRAM

| | Exercise | Sets | Repetitions |
|---|---|---|---|
| Monday: | Bench Press | 5 | 1–5 |
| | Cleans | 5 | 1–5 |
| | Squats | 5 | 1–5 |
| | Biceps Curls | 3 | 10 |
| | French Curls | 3 | 10 |
| | Pullovers | 3 | 10 |
| | Situps (weights) | 3 | 10 |
| Wednesday: | Incline Press | 5 | 5 |
| | Snatch | 5 | 1–5 |
| | Squats | 5 | 5 |
| | Dumbbell Curls | 3 | 10 |
| | Bar Dips (weights) | 3 | 5 |
| | Pullups (weights) | 3 | 5–10 |
| | Situps | 3 | 25–50 |

| | Exercise | Sets | Repetitions |
|---|---|---|---|
| Friday: | Bench Press | 5 | 5 |
| | High Pulls | 5 | 5 |
| | Squats | 5 | 1–5 |
| | Biceps Curls | 3 | 10 |
| | French Curls | 3 | 10 |
| | Pullovers | 3 | 10 |
| | Situps | 3 | 25 |

## INSTANT REPLAY

1. Strength and power are important for sports.
2. You should strength train two to three days per week.
3. Strength is specific. You should train many areas of your body.
4. You can develop with or without equipment. To reach high levels of strength, you probably should join a health club or train at a local college.
5. Strength training will not develop a significant amount of cardiovascular endurance.
6. Do your exercises with good technique to avoid injury.

# CHAP7TER

# DEVELOPING FLEXIBILITY

"**C**ome on Fahey, touch those toes; you look like an old man," yelled my college coach, Bob Lualhati.

"Give me a break, coach. My muscles feel like strands of aluminum foil, and they won't stretch any more."

I've never been very flexible. In college I was a discus thrower, and my training consisted of throwing, heavy weight lifting, and some running. When the coach tried to get the "heavies" to stretch, we would hide behind the pole vault pit. Instead of trying to increase my meager flexibility, I was more concerned about saving face around the ultra-flexible hurdlers and high jumpers.

After my competitive discus throwing days ended, I soon learned the cost of being inflexible. As I tried a variety of sports, I became sore in new places and developed a rash of injuries. Around that time sports-oriented physicians and athletic trainers began to stress the importance of flexibility exercises as a preventive measure against injuries. I began slowly, but little by little I developed increased mobility in many of the joints of my body. Those aches and pains disappeared.

Several professional football teams have substantially reduced their rate of injuries by emphasizing flexibility exercises in their programs. I think it's a good idea if you regularly incorporate stretching exercises into your training schedule. You are less likely to get hurt, and the increased range of motion may help your sports performance. Lack of joint mobility is a common characteristic of aging. If you consistently work the parts of your body through a complete range of motion, you can maintain joint mobility throughout your lifetime. Even those aches and pains you sometimes feel when you get up in the morning may be less severe when you regularly practice these kinds of exercises.

## WHAT DETERMINES HOW FLEXIBLE YOU ARE?

To a large extent, your activities determine how flexible you are. When you regularly repeat movement, your body seems to adjust and moves toward an optimum flexibility. When learning a skill, flexibility will probably mean little in determining your performance; but as you become more proficient, that extra range of motion may make a difference.

Muscle cells are held together in bundles by connective tissue and fascia. Fascia and connective tissue blend into tendons that hold muscle to bone. Muscle tissue itself has no ability to stretch; it shortens when it contracts, but it returns to its normal length after the contraction. Flexibility exercises affect connective tissue the most. There is also some effect on tendons, ligaments, joint capsules, and muscle fascia.

The nervous system is probably the most important factor that determines your flexibility. Your muscles, joints, tendons, and ligaments have a very prolific nerve supply. Special nerves called stretch receptors tell your muscles how far they're being stretched. Stretch receptors are important in protecting your muscles from being stretched too far. They are involved in maintaining the balance that must exist in body movements. They aid in the contraction-relaxation cycle of muscles in activities such as running.

Your muscle size also affects joint mobility. Large biceps (upper arm muscles) will get in the way when the forearm is attempting to move throughout the range of motion. To many people, large muscles may be more important than flexibility. You should seek a balance between muscle size and flexibility.

Strength and power are important for tennis and other sports.

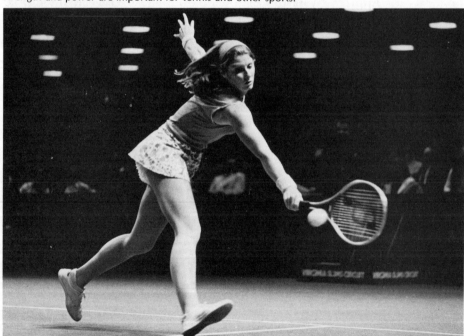

# GUIDELINES FOR STRETCHING

1. Flexibility exercises are not competitive. Increase your range of motion gradually. Overdoing this kind of exercise can lead to injury.
2. Do not bounce when you stretch. Bouncing may cause small tears in your muscles. In addition, bouncing may stimulate the stretch receptors, causing your muscles to tighten up. Your stretching movements should be done gently and gradually. Flinging-type stretching exercises may also result in stretch tears that appear in or below the skin.
3. On cold days it is particularly important to stretch adequately before exercising. Studies have shown flexibility to decrease 10 to 20 percent when joint temperatures are lowered.
4. Relax as much as possible during stretching exercises. There is a direct relationship between state of mind and muscle tension. Relaxation is also important for fluid, graceful performance.
5. Practice your flexibility exercises regularly. Increased joint mobility can only be attained by systematic effort.
6. Stretch before and after exercise. Stretching before training will help prevent injuries, while stretching afterward will help keep muscle soreness to a minimum.
7. Flexibility is not an end in itself. You must incorporate an increased range of motion into your sports techniques. Increased flexibility should not be gained at the expense of speed.
8. Stretch until you feel a noticeable "pull" in your muscles. Hold that position for 15 to 30 seconds. Relax and then repeat the exercise.
9. Do not cheat on your exercises. Do the exercises as shown in the photographs. However, do not overstretch. As soon as you feel pain, do not try to stretch any further until the pain subsides.
10. Include exercises from all categories of stretching. Mix up the order of the exercises. Do one for the legs, another for the back, and then go back to the legs. Don't do all the exercises for one body part consecutively.

# Flexibility Exercises

Flexibility exercises can be grouped into four categories:

1. Waist and back
2. Hip and thigh
3. Shoulder
4. Feet and lower legs

Choose at least two exercises from each category. Stretch before and after exercise. You may find it helpful to do a few of these movements when you get up in the morning. They may help you get your day started. Try to do the exercises according to the instructions. Remember, stretch to a point where you feel a pulling sensation in your muscles; hold that position for 20 to 30 seconds; relax and repeat the movement at least once more.

## WAIST AND BACK EXERCISES

1. Waist Benders
   Keeping your legs straight, bend forward at your waist and extend your arms toward your feet until you feel a stretch. Hold the stretch for 20 to 30 seconds. Bend your knees (to protect your back), and return to a normal standing position. Repeat at least once. You will feel this one in your lower back and in your hamstring muscles.
2. Sitting Stretches
   In sitting position with feet about six inches apart, reach and grab your legs as far down as possible. Try to move your head toward your knees. Hold that position for 20 to 30 seconds. Relax and then repeat. This exercise is good for the back and hamstrings.
3. Back Rollers
   In seated position, bend your knees and hold them with your hands. Pull your knees toward your chest and gently roll backwards. Hold this position about 30 seconds. Relax and repeat. This is a good one for your lower back.
4. Advanced Back Rollers
   From seated position, bring knees to your chest and continue to rock back until your feet touch the floor behind you. Hold for 30 seconds and repeat. This is a lot harder than it looks, so don't try it right away.

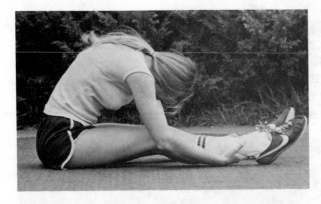

Sitting stretch

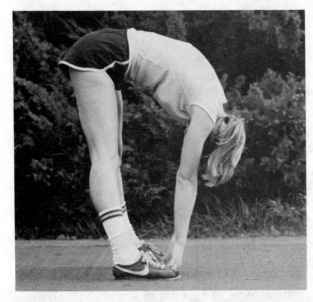

Waist bender

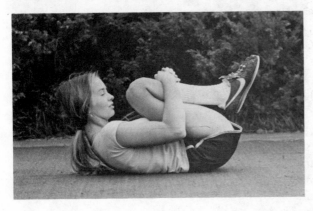

Back roller

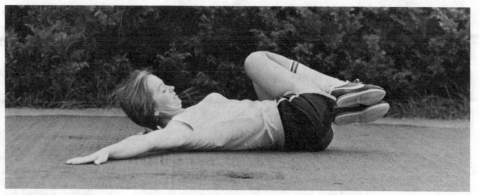

Twister

5. Twisters
   Lie on your back with your knees bent. Spread your arms out to provide support. Keeping your knees together, turn them both to the ground on the right and then on the left. Repeat five to ten times.

## HIP AND THIGH

There are obvious overlaps between waist-and-back and hip-and-leg stretching exercises. Classifications are used for convenience.

1. Groin stretch
   In seated position, put the soles of your feet together and gently press the inside of your knees with your elbows. Hold the stretch for 20 to 30 seconds. Relax and repeat. The groin is an area that is often injured in high-intensity sports, such as basketball and tennis.
2. Hurdler Stretch: Quadriceps (muscles on front of thigh)
   In sitting position, put one leg forward and bend the other backward so that you are leaning on your shin. Lean back so that you feel a pull in the muscles on the front of your thigh. Hold for 20 to 30 seconds. Relax and repeat. Switch positions and work on the other leg.
3. Hurdler Stretch: Hamstrings (muscles on back of thigh)
   Assume hurdler stretch position described for the last exercise. Bend forward until you feel a pull in the back of your leg. Relax and repeat. Switch positions and work on the other leg.

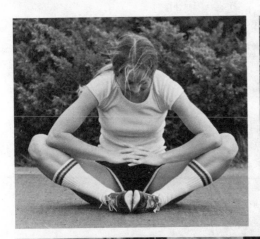
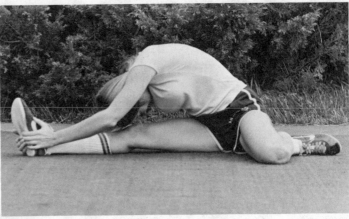

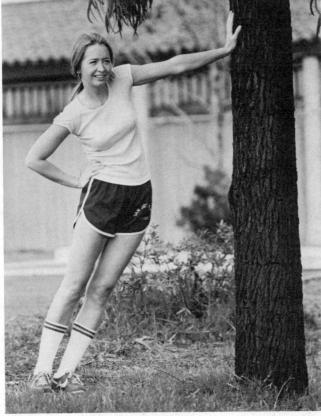

*Left above:* Groin stretch
*Right above:* Hurdler stretch
*Left:* Hip stretch

### 4. Hip Stretches

Stand about 18 inches from a wall or lamp post. Lean on the wall with your hand or forearm and push your hips inward. Hold for 20 to 30 seconds, relax, and repeat the exercise. Switch sides and stretch the other hip. This one is great for preventing sore hips that sometimes arise from jogging.

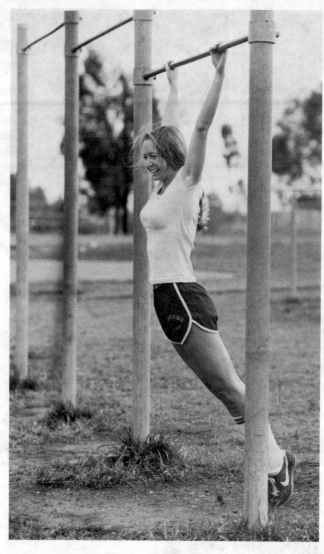

Shoulder bender

## SHOULDERS

The shoulder joint is constructed to provide maximum mobility. Many aches and pains in this area are caused by loss of range of motion through disuse or from chronic exercise of the shoulders in a restricted way (improper weight training techniques, for example.)

1. Shoulder Benders
   Place your hands shoulder width apart on a bar or wall. Keeping your legs straight, let your upper body hang down as

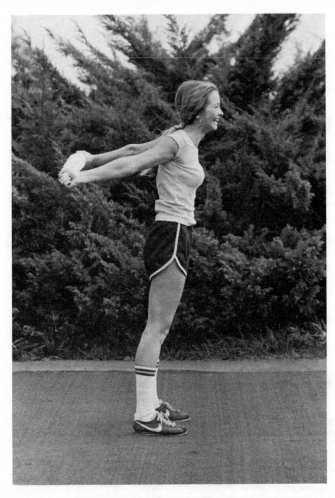

Shoulder circles with a towel

you keep your knees locked. Feel the stretch in your shoulders and upper back. Hold for 20 to 30 seconds. Relax and repeat the exercise.

2. Shoulder Circles With A Towel

Hold both ends of a towel, with hands a little wider than shoulder width apart. Raise your hands over your head and continue rotating your arms until you're holding the towel behind your back. As you become more flexible, grasp the towel with your hands closer together. This is a favorite exercise of Olympic weight lifters and is great for increasing shoulder flexibility.

3. Wings

   Hold your arms out in front of you; then move them horizontally until you feel a stretch in your chest muscles. Hold the stretch for 20 to 30 seconds. Relax and repeat.

4. Shoulder Shrugs

   Shrug your shoulders upward. Hold for five seconds. Then rotate them forward very slowly. Repeat this five to ten times.

## FEET AND LOWER LEG EXERCISES

Foot and ankle exercises are extremely important for preventing aches and pains and injury. If you would take a few minutes each day to do a few of these simple exercises, you could avoid problems that sometimes can take months or even years to clear up.

1. Achilles Tendon Stretch

   Lean far enough away from a wall so that you are on your toes with your heels off the ground. You should feel a stretch in your calf muscles and in your Achilles tendons. A variation of

Achilles tendon stretch

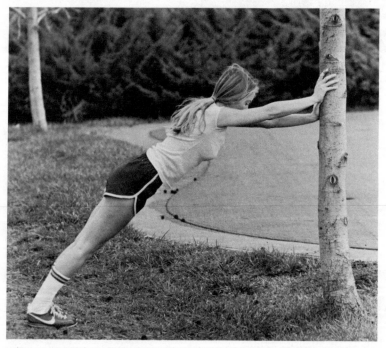

this exercise is to stretch one leg at a time. This exercise is a must for the jogger.

2. Shin Stretchers

   In a kneeling position, place your feet so that the tops are facing the floor. Gently sit back on your heels so that you feel a stretch in your shins and top part of your foot. This is a great exercise for preventing shin splints.

3. Footsies

   Work your feet through a variety of ranges of motion. Flex and extend your toes and twist your feet inward and outward. This is a good exercise if you have sore feet in the morning. Do this exercise before you get out of bed.

There are many other possible stretching exercises. The principles are the same for any of them. These are just a few of the most popular.

Yoga is a system of exercises that is excellent for developing flexibility. Most of the postures are held for a sustained period of time, so there is little risk of injury if you don't push yourself too far. A description of yoga exercises is beyond the scope of this book. As with any other types of exercise, yoga makes a contribution to total fitness, but it doesn't do the whole thing. Yoga has an air of mysticism about it that may make you believe you're involved in some sort of "total experience." However, yoga will not improve your endurance, strength, or skill required for sports. It's great, but it's only part of your fitness program.

Make flexibility training an important part of your preparation for sports. If you put in just ten minutes a day, you will see noticeable changes within a matter of weeks. Don't go too fast. Increase your range of motion gradually.

## INSTANT REPLAY

1. Your activities determine the extent of your flexibility.
2. Increase your flexibility gradually.
3. Don't bounce when you stretch.
4. Don't cheat on your exercises. Do your flexibility exercises with good technique.

CHAP8TER

THE MAIN EVENT

I started skiing as a sophomore in high school at the age of 15. On my first trip, I borrowed my father's cousin's boots, winter clothing, and skis. The skis were 210 centimeters long and had wooden edges. They had bear claw bindings, which acted as a vise to hold the boots firmly in place. On my first day I climbed up a small hill and attempted to "ski" to the bottom without killing myself. The next day I decided to give the rope tow a try. This made the process much easier and skiing a lot more fun. Although that first winter I made only one trip to the mountains, I became totally enamored of the sport.

During the off season I became obsessed with skiing. I read ski magazines, went to countless sport and ski shops, and watched ski movies. It was the ski movies that proved to be my undoing. They showed people like Stein Erickson gliding down steep, powdery mountainsides with ease. They made it look easy. "Anyone can do that," I told myself. "All you have to do is point your skis down the hill and make S turns all the way to the bottom." I imagined myself a good skier. I soon forgot the reality of those long boards and the rope tow. I was a skier. I, too, could easily glide to the bottom of the steepest ski run.

Winter came once again, and I was ready. I rode the chairlift to the top of KT-22, an expert ski run at Squaw Valley. I showed no fear, because after all I was a proficient skier. I got off the chair and in front of me was a ledge overlooking a steep face. I paused for a minute and then proceeded to jump over the edge. I flew through the air and by some miracle landed on my feet. But then the truth caught up with me—I was the same skier who had been on the rope tow the season before. I didn't know how to turn and was now racing out of control on one of the steepest runs in America. I fell; hat, poles, and goggles were strewn about the mountain, and my mouth filled with snow. My vivid imagination had almost caused me to be maimed for life. I somehow made it down the hill and back to the rope tow. I decided to take a ski lesson and begin again, this time the right way. "Bend-z-knees, five dollars please."

Learning a skill is never easy. There are right ways and wrong ways. There are sports scientists who specialize in the optimal way of learning sports and movement skill. This area of specialization is called motor learning. These people have developed general principles that will help you improve your performance.

## MOTOR LEARNING HAS NOTHING TO DO WITH CARS

The efficiency of your movements determines how well you will perform a skill. Let's say, for example, you wish to hit a tennis ball over a net. In your mind you already have an image of the manner in which you plan to do this. If you are a skilled tennis player, then your actual movement will be similar to your mental image. If, on the other hand, you are a beginning player, there will be much wasted motion, and your actual motion may be a lot different than your mental picture. Learning a sports skill involves developing a consistency between your mental image of a movement and your actual performance.

Most movement and sports skills are learned. For success in sports, you have to make your movements become almost like a reflex. Reflex sports performance comes only from hours of practice. It's most important to learn the correct technique early. If you constantly practice a faulty technique, you may develop bad habits that you never shake. Develop the fundamentals of a sport—then work on the razzle-dazzle stuff.

You may not be capable of using the techniques of professional and Olympic athletes. Learn techniques that are appropriate to your present level of ability. Top athletes have extremely well-developed speed, power, and flexibility. A technique that works for them may not work for you. Take lessons from an expert, preferably one who knows how to teach and can lead you through a learning program suitable for a beginner.

A major premise of this book is that physical fitness requires a number of physical experiences. You need strength, speed, endurance, and flexibility. Current research indicates that the more movement experiences you have, the better you will be able to adjust to new sports and exercises. So, if you have a sports-oriented lifestyle, you have a better chance to learn new skills.

## PRACTICE SESSIONS

If you want to play up to expectations, then you have to practice. Break down your game and analyze your strengths and weaknesses. Work on those aspects of the technique that are going to make the most difference. In tennis, for example, if you can't serve, then working on a slicing backhand is pretty ridiculous. Work on your serve first. When working on a movement, overlearn it. Work on a skill until it becomes like a reflex. Develop skills that you can count on. When you do that, you will have the "winning edge."

When beginning to learn a skill, it's best to have a number of short practice sessions rather than one or two long ones. Long sessions lead to fatigue, and you learn little when you are tired. This is especially true when your level of physical fitness is low.

Similar sports may interfere with the learning process, a phenomenon called negative transfer. Tennis, for example, requires you keep your wrist relatively firm. Badminton requires a lot of wrist action. One sport may disrupt your learning the other. It's best to learn similar sports one at a time. Learn one skill and then another, and you'll have fewer problems.

Sports should be practiced at realistic speed. "Slow motion" practice may be valuable for gaining a mental picture of a skill but will do little to improve your performance. Practice a skill at the same speed as in a game. Accuracy is important as well. If a sport requires accuracy, then practice accuracy. You should practice speed and accuracy early in the learning process for the best results.

People differ in the rate they learn sports skills. You can maximize your learning by following some simple guidelines. Constantly assess your performance. Don't practice haphazardly. Think about what you are doing correctly and what needs work. Concentrate! Your mind and body work like a computer in many ways. Eliminate your mistakes and take advantage of your strong points. Work to make your skills automatic. Your goal is to direct your attention to the game rather than to the details. Make the skill as simple as possible. If your movements are simple, then there are fewer chances of mistakes.

## MENTAL IMAGES

Divers and gymnasts always form a mental picture of their movements. You can do this for any sport. When you have developed an image in your mind, it's much easier to zero in on efficient performance. When you are lying in bed, think about how you are going to perform in a sport. Picture yourself going through the entire movement pattern. Develop a positive image of yourself. Picture yourself moving gracefully, performing perfectly. If you do this consistently, you will become more like your mental image.

I can't overestimate the importance or necessity of psyche. If you can feel what you're going to do, chances are you will do it. Perry

O'Brien, the great shotputter of the 1950's, used to dream about his technique. He would often wake up in the middle of the night and work on some point of technique he had dreamed about. When you think about technique a great deal, it will become second nature to you. You will learn to feel it.

"Paralysis by analysis" occurs when your sports performance deteriorates because you have overintellectualized about your technique. Although most sports skills are made up of many components, overemphasizing parts of a technique may result in interrupted, jerky movements. Efficient movements are smooth and appear effortless. As a young discus thrower, I stared for hours at loop films of my boyhood idol, Al Oerter, the renowned American Olympian. A loop film is a sports technique film that runs continuously. Watching Oerter helped me form a mental image of the technique I was trying to accomplish. Although he was generating tremendous power, his movements looked effortless. The only way you can put it all together is to combine all the components of your technique into a fluid movement. Academic understanding of a sport is great, but if you can't feel the movements, you'll never become fluid and smooth.

Videotape is an electronic way of matching your performance to your mental image. Many colleges and teachers of various sports now routinely use videotape for lessons. This gives you immediate feedback on what you are doing wrong. If you can feel a movement, this is better than verbalizing it. You can talk all day about arm positions and leg movements, but if you can't feel it, it simply won't sink in.

## GOALS

The toughest part of making the transition to an activity-oriented lifestyle is developing a positive mental attitude. Your goals should reflect self-improvement. Say to yourself, "I can be better." You can always be a little better than you are now. Forget about quantum improvements and concentrate on short-term gains.

Success breeds success. Develop series of short-term goals. Achieve one, then establish another. Don't set your goals so high that you will fail. However, don't sell yourself short either. In the movie *Rocky* a small-time fighter gets a chance at the world championship. His goal becomes staying in the ring with the champ. If he had set his goal higher, he might have won; but he might also have quit in frustration.

I have stated several times that the beginning jock is really no different than the professional jock or the Olympian. All jocks are involved in a process of enjoying sports and physical activity; all are trying to improve themselves. Success at sports, as in anything else, requires sustained concentration. With time you can improve your skills in any sport. Learn the required skills one at a time. Practice them until they become smooth and until you develop the ability to use them effectively.

Few things are more satisfying than mastering a skill. You can do it if you just make a small commitment. The choice is yours. In the *Iliad* of Homer, Achilles is offered the choice of a long and uneventful life or a short and glorious one. Your choice is similar, with several exceptions. If you choose the active, sports-oriented life, your years will be exciting, fun, fulfilling, and perhaps even longer. If you choose the sedentary life, your years will probably be duller, and you may be less healthy.

## TYING IT TOGETHER

If you had the stamina and the resources, you could spend every waking hour playing sports. You could play golf in the morning; go for a run at lunch; play a little tennis in the afternoon; and lift some weights at night. When you got bored you could fly down to South America for some summer skiing. Most of us don't have the time or the money.

Figure out how much time you have available. If you say "no time," then you are depriving yourself of an important part of life. Working people have five basic times for exercise:

1. Before work
2. Lunch time
3. After work
4. Weekends
5. Vacations

Give yourself some of this time. Write down a schedule for yourself, and go out and have fun. For example:

Monday     6:00 a.m.   — Jogging and Stretching
             9:00 p.m.   — Racquetball
Tuesday    12:00 Noon — Strength Training

| Wednesday | 12:00 Noon | — Tennis |
| | 7:00 p.m. | — Stationary Bike |
| Thursday | 12:00 Noon | — Strength Training |
| Friday | 6:00 a.m. | — Interval Training |
| Saturday | 10:00 a.m. | — Jog with family or friend |
| Sunday | All Day | — Hike |

On your vacation, go to a place with some opportunities for physical activity. There are countless things you can do. Go to the beach; go backpacking; play tennis; go to a sports camp for adults. I went to a summer ski camp a few summers ago and had a great time.

If you don't know how to play many sports, learn some. Write down about five sports you want to learn and "go to it." You will gain enough skill to have fun rapidly. Fun is the key to the whole thing. If you're having fun, it doesn't matter that you're not a world champion. Give this lifestyle a chance, and you will get the health benefits of exercise and have a lot more fun at the same time.

## BEGINNING YOUR EXERCISE PROGRAM

### How do I get Started?

It's easy to get started: First, find out what you want from an exercise program. Sit down and write out everything you hope to gain. For example:

1. Lose 10 pounds and look better in a swim suit
2. Improve fitness for skiing
3. Play tennis better
4. Learn how to scuba dive
5. Improve health

Second, figure out what you will have to do to achieve your objectives:

1. To lose 10 pounds and look better in a swim suit, you are going to have to modify your diet and increase your training time. Some firming exercises might also help.
2. Skiing requires strength, quickness, flexibility, and stamina.

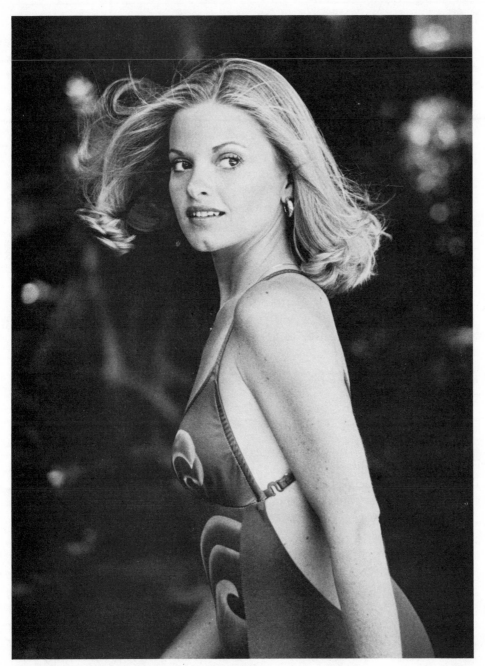

Looking good in a bathing suit takes a lot of work.

Also, improved skill makes the sport a lot easier—maybe a few lessons would help speed things along.

3. For tennis you will need to develop some specific skills. Instead of going out and just hitting the ball, maybe some drills would be helpful. Learn a few shots that will consistently put your opponent away. Develop a serve with a little juice in it. Learn that cross-court backhand that you admire so much. These shots require systematic training.

4. Scuba diving requires a certificate. You will need to take lessons from a certified instructor. A trip to your local college or dive shop should do the trick.

5. To improve your health and possibly offer yourself some protection against heart disease, you have to set aside some time for regular endurance exercise, at least three to five times per week.

Third, after you have figured out what's involved in meeting your goals, set up a plan. As a "Total Jock" you are going to need a program that prepares you for a lot of sports. Make a commitment—choose regular times to exercise. Find out where you can get professional instruction.

Success in a new sport requires

1. Developing good fundamentals
2. Purchasing the best equipment you can afford

I can't overstate the importance of developing good fundamentals. If you are well-schooled in the basics, they become instinctive even if you haven't played in a long time. Good performance requires consistency—the most consistent player is the one with the best fundamentals. Developing good skills is sometimes boring and tedious, but the results are consistent play. Good equipment is important in any sport. Beginners in many sports often have miserable experiences because they usually use cheap equipment. They spend as much time trying to compensate for their poor equipment as they do learning the sport. If you take a little time to select good equipment and get some good advice, you will have a good time. In a sport like scuba diving, cheap equipment can kill you. Sixty feet under the water is no place to have your regulator go out on you. Good equipment can only help your performance. When buying equipment for any sport, ask around. Talk to people who play the sport. Don't ask the salespeople in big department

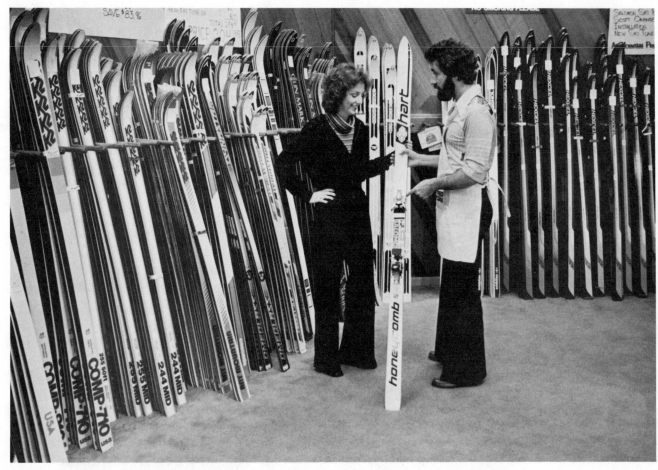

Buy your equipment from an expert.

stores—they may not know much about the equipment. Specialty sports stores are often a good bet.

Finally, make up your mind that sports and exercise are an important part of your lifestyle. Don't try to do it all today—you have the rest of your life.

## Do I Need to Buy Any Special Clothes?

You can spend a tremendous amount of money on sports clothes. For running you can buy a pair of shorts and a T-shirt for a few dollars or fancy sweat suits for lots of dollars. Clothes for any sport should be practical. If you find a pair of running shorts on sale that tear easily, you've lost your bargain.

For sports requiring high levels of exertion, such as running, you should make sure that the fabric will allow you to dissipate heat. Dr. Harmon Brown (Olympic team physician and coach) and I found that people training with sweat suits on a moderately hot day raised their body temperatures above 104 degrees. Improper clothes can certainly make your exercise program miserable. I always shudder to see beginning runners wearing full-length jeans. On cold days, too much clothing may also be a problem. If your exercise is intermittent, such as downhill skiing, have a warm top you can put on during rest periods. Take off the top when you're working hard.

Clothes are very important to many people for psychological reasons. Don't get so bogged down with expensive clothes that you can't afford the sport. Remember, the person in Aspen wearing a pair of jeans is going to have more fun than the person stuck at home with a $200 ski suit he can't afford.

## How do I Choose a Pair of Shoes?

Make sure your shoes fit. No matter what the sport, you won't enjoy yourself if your feet hurt. The shoes you buy should be appropriate to the activity. You can't satisfactorily use a running shoe for tennis or

Choose the shoe that's best for you.

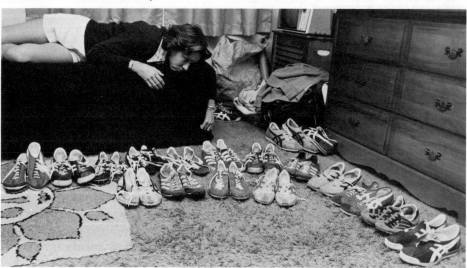

racquetball and vice versa. Use your judgement; don't let a salesperson sell you something you won't be happy with. Don't fall for the old line, "Oh, don't worry, they'll fit after they've stretched a bit." Consult people involved in the sport. They can usually steer you away from the ripoffs and direct you toward something that's best for you.

Shoe design has evolved from a hit-or-miss proposition to a real science. Biomechanics laboratories have identified what factors are important in running shoes by using high-speed film and sophisticated electronics to analyze runners. They've found the initial shock occurs at the heel and progresses toward the outer edge of the foot. The foot rotates inward as shock is absorbed by the ball of the foot. Forward energy is then required as the runner pushes off. Shoe selection should take into consideration the forces involved in running. A good shoe should provide adequate support and cushioning at the heel. A firm arch support is needed to aid in transferring your weight to the ball of your foot. You need good cushioning in the front part of the shoe, particularly the outer edge. Finally, your shoe should provide good flexibility and traction at the front of the sole for your forward drive.

Each October, *Runner's World* magazine provides an analysis of the top running shoes on the market. Shoes are judged in a scientific laboratory and by a panel of experts. The laboratory tests include flexibility, impact response, and sole wear. You can use this evaluation to help you choose the shoe that's best for you. Remember, if your shoes don't fit correctly, their top rating doesn't matter. The best shoes of most companies are finely crafted and should meet the requirements of all but the fussiest runners. Shop around. Try on a variety of shoes and then make up your mind.

Shoes for court games have different requirements. Tennis, racquetball, badminton, and basketball involve quick changes of direction. The shoes must provide lateral support to give protection against ankle injury and blisters. The shoe should be thinner than jogging shoes and minimize slippage of your foot. They should also provide good arch support. Court shoes generally have less flexibility in the soles.

Choosing shoes and boots for other sports is no less complicated. Again, seek the advice of experts. Many boots have specialized purposes. Ski boots, for example, are designed with the skill level of the skier in mind. Racing boots have a pronounced forward lean and are extremely stiff. They are inappropriate for people who have to stand in lift lines and might like to stand up straight some time. Boots used for climbing are usually too stiff for backpacking, even though they may look alike. Specialized magainzes such as *Ski, Backpacker,* and *Climbing Magazine* sometimes offer equipment analysis. Such consumer information is helpful for selecting products in your price range and level of ability and experience. Shoes are usually the most important piece of equipment for any sport. Choose them wisely; nobody likes sore feet.

## What Is a Training Diary?

One of the best ways to keep track of your exercise program is by keeping a training diary. Most successful athletes write down the progress they're making in their workouts. A diary helps you to be systematic in your program and enables you to better measure your progress. Twenty-nine-year-old Bruce Kennedy, national javelin champion, has kept such a diary since he was 12 years old. He can systematically evaluate which methods have led to success and which have been a waste of time. He doesn't have to guess about his training; it's written down for him. A training diary will help you in several ways:

1. By writing down your workout for the day, you will be more likely to have a thorough program. The diary provides a goal incentive. If you enter in your diary that today you will run three miles, play racquetball, and lift weights, you'll probably do it! Completing your assigned workout is like fulfilling a promise to yourself.
2. The training diary allows you to improve systematically. Training for most people is a hit-or-miss proposition. They go out to the track or health club and do what they feel like doing. If they are ambitious, they may do a lot of work—sometimes too much. Usually, however, they don't do enough. By keeping a record, you can easily see when it's time to pour it on.
3. The training diary allows you to chart your progress. You can see when you are improving. With time, it's sometimes difficult to monitor your progress. It's hard to imagine yourself out of shape and inept after you have become fit and skilled.

The following is an example of a page from a training diary:

**Training Diary of SALLY JOCK**
**Date: 8/17/80**

---

1. Health Status: Feel great. No aches and pains.
   Body weight: 125 pounds

2. Flexibility Exercises: "Total Jock" flexibility exercises
for ten minutes.

3. Endurance Exercises: Ran three miles at the Canyon (up
and down hills). Time about 25
minutes.
Exercise heart rate about 165 beats per minute.

4. Sports: Played racquetball with John over at the club.
Wiped him out!

5. Speed Exercises: None

6. Goals For Month: Begin conditioning for ski season.
Join volleyball league at the college.


## Do I Need to Get a Medical Examination?

If you are young and healthy, the physical exam you get every couple of years is probably sufficient. Your chances of developing serious problems are remote. However, if you're over 35 years old or have health problems (obesity, smoking, high blood pressure, etc.), you should see your physician before beginning an exercise program. Exercise can be dangerous if you're out of shape and haven't taken care of yourself. Your medical exam should ideally include an electrocardiogram conducted at rest and during exercise.

If you don't have a physician, it's best to get one who understands exercise. Try to find a doctor who is a jock. Inquire at your local medical society or medical school. A team physician of a high school or college can often tell you which doctors in the community are interested in sports medicine. Exercise training is a science in itself. Although there are many physicians who know a great deal about exercise physiology, there are others who know little. Medical schools spend little time on exercise physiology. An uninformed physician won't be able to provide you with much advice about your program. Usually doctors who exercise themselves are your best bet.


## Where Can I Take a Treadmill Test?

The treadmill test is one of the best noninvasive measures of assessing the health of your heart. This test can accurately assess your physical fitness and oxygen consumption (max mets). It can be used to determine the optimal workout pace for your training program. In Chapter 4, I have included several tests that will approximate the results of the treadmill. However, the treadmill enables the precise measurement of your capacity in a controlled environment. If you are going to have a heart problem, it is better to have it in a clinical atmosphere where trained people can help you. If you choose to measure your own capacity with the tests in this book, I cannot emphasize enough the importance of first completing the preliminary conditioning exercises.

Many physicians, universities, and private companies are set up to provide exercise stress tests at a modest fee. I would suggest you contact the physical education department of a large university in your area or your local medical society. Many places that offer treadmill tests also have an associated adult fitness program. If you are just starting to exercise, a supervised program is often your best bet.

## Am I Too Old?

There was storm surf at Santa Cruz. Fifteen- to twenty-foot waves crashed up on the beach. Down the face of a wave plummeted two black bodies. One, a seal frolicking in the waves. The other, 60-year-old Bob Titchenel, clad in a full wetsuit to protect him from the freezing winter water. Titchenel is a great all-round athlete. He played professional football for 15 years, and then had an active career as a football coach. He won major California body surfing championships in his 50's. He plays most sports better than people one-third his age. Sure, Titchenel is exceptional, but his lifestyle keeps him that way.

If you're older, you have to start more slowly. However, you can reach higher levels of performance regardless of your age. Dr. Fred Kasch, an exercise physiologist who has studied middle-aged men and women, has found that in some ways regular exercise retards the aging process. Metabolic capacity and muscle mass, which usually decline drastically during middle age, actually improved when men and women remained on a jogging program. Ponce de Leon didn't have to search for the fountain of youth—all he had to do was train.

Larry Lewis, who died of cancer in 1974, ran five miles a day when he was over 100 years old. In my laboratory I see many men and women in their 40's, 50's, and 60's who put most teenagers to shame. No matter what your age, if you consistently train and try to improve, you will reach a pretty high level of fitness.

## Where Can I Receive Instruction?

One of the best places to receive sports instruction is in a class. Take a class at your local high school, college, or recreation department. They have classes in everything from rock climbing and white water rafting to hang gliding and conditioning. These classes are inexpensive and provide you with the opportunity to meet people with the same interests and level of ability.

Private lessons, although expensive, may be more valuable if you are trying to refine a particular technique. Private lessons sometimes enable you to get better quality instruction with fewer hassles—but you pay for it.

Instruction of some kind is the best way to begin a new sport. Professional instruction is always better than learning from your friends. A pro knows how to teach, as well as what to teach. A person with great athletic skill may not be able to translate movements into words and/or tolerate a beginner's ineptness.

## Is Competition Important?

Two men, drenched in sweat, faced each other with the resolve of knights doing battle. A ball careened into the air. One of the men dove for it, crashing against the floor. The ball was smashed by the other man at an angle toward the front wall; it bounced—once, twice, three times, and then rolled to a stop. Was this the national racquetball championship where life itself appeared to be on the line? No, it was the warm-ups of the Fahey family racquetball championship. At stake—the family champion perpetual trophy.

My brother and I are perhaps two of the worst racquetball players in America. Yet to us our weekly racquetball games are very important. We went to a trophy shop and had a small plaque made up as a symbol of victory for the current winner of our tournament. Each week the winner gets to proudly display the trophy in his home. This little gimmick keeps the games interesting and fun. You don't have to buy a trophy. You can use an old shoe, a T-shirt, or whatever you have handy.

Formal competitions are available in many sports for people of all levels of ability. Mary is a born-again housewife turned marathon runner. She runs over 70 miles a week and seems to enter competitive races about once a month. She is far from being a speed burner, but she

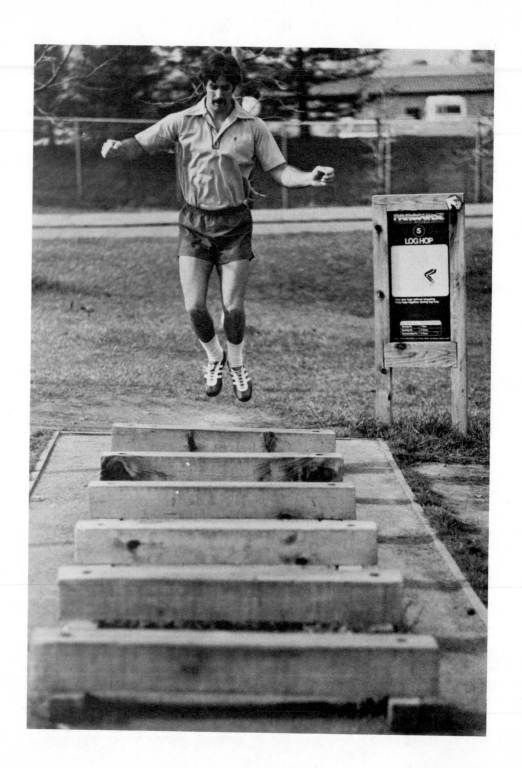

loves the process of training for those competitions. She commented, "I'm getting to the point where I hate running in these races—they interrupt my training and prevent me from running the mileage I would like." She is involved in the sports process. Competition was the vehicle that got her into the whole thing. However, it's the process that's important to her now.

I have friends who have been discus throwers and shotputters for over 20 years. They are past their peak and have little chance of ever making the Olympic team. Why do they continue? They are in love with the process of sport.

Competition can be a means of joining the sporting life. This competition can range from a golf match between two duffers to the highest level of sport. The essence is exactly the same.

## How Can I Get My Family Involved?

I have found that people who meet resistance from their families about their exercise program don't follow it for very long. If you make your regular exercise outings fun, your family will look forward to sports participation. You have to take into consideration each person's abilities and expectations. If you try to force someone to be competitive and he feels uncomfortable, he will stop training with you.

There are many family-oriented activities you can do. Skiing, horseback riding, volleyball, hiking, swimming, body surfing, jogging, and badminton are just a few. Many cities now have par courses in their parks. A par course is a jogging trail with exercise stations at various intervals. These jogging trails are springing up all over the country and are generally a great success. Thousands of people use these courses every day. The par course has become a regular outing for many families.

Many sports have family activities built into their competitive structure. Track and field and swimming have always been strong in this area. Now, it's possible to get the family involved in the competitive aspects of skiing, tennis, soccer, and sailing. Even young children can get into the act. I've seen six-year-olds compete in 10,000 meter runs. I think as long as it's fun and you don't pressure your child, he or she can do almost anything. Remember, a six-year-old is not a miniature adult. Keep

The par course: a jogging trail with exercise stations.

it fun and your family will develop positive attitudes toward sports and exercise.

## Where Can I Meet People to Train With?

Meeting people through sports is important:

1. New friends may be essential for breaking into sports requiring expensive equipment or specialized skill.
2. Friends make participation in sports more enjoyable.

I had wanted to learn to sail a Hobie Cat for many years. A Hobie Cat is a catamaran sailboat whose speed can exceed 25 miles per hour on a windy day. When you really get going, one side of the boat will rise out of the water so that you're sailing on only one hull. The problem was I didn't own a boat and didn't know anyone who did. One day at Lake Tahoe I got into a conversation with some Hobie owners, and before I knew it, I was sailing. With the many sports possibilities available, each jock will have had a variety of experiences. You may be a hang gliding enthusiast but know nothing about sky diving. Someone else can help you get started. People you meet on the trail may be able to direct you to a lake with great fishing. A new opponent may teach you some new tricks or provide you with new perspectives on your abilities. Association with people is one of the joys of a sports-oriented lifestyle. People will help you branch out in your sports skills—either by providing you with new experiences or by sharpening your technique.

Structured situations are often best for meeting new training partners. Exercise and sports classes allow you to meet people with similar abilities and interests. Classes also offer the opportunity for you to sample various activities without great investments of time or money. Various types of health clubs may provide a socially conducive atmosphere. Many clubs provide opportunities for competition in racquetball, tennis, and weight lifting. You don't have to be King Kong to join club tournaments. Competitions are offered for many levels of ability for men, women, and children. Many clubs have even gone as far as providing bar service for their clientele.

I think the most important benefit I've received from my association with sports has been the friends I've met along the way. People are an important part of this active lifestyle. Telling stories about that great ski run or that winning shot that just hit the line is half the fun of being a jock. When you're a jock the active life engulfs your body and soul.